WARD LOCK

FAMILY HEALTH GUIDE

ASTHMA &
ALLERGIES

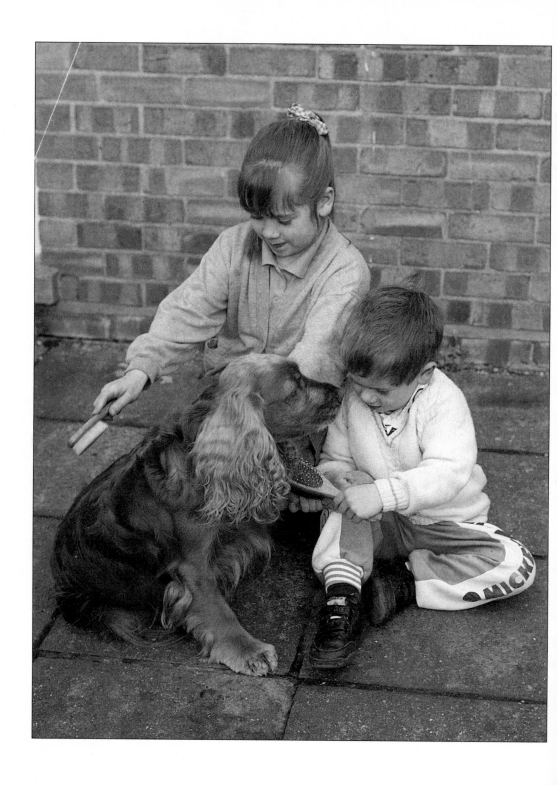

WARD LOCK

FAMILY HEALTH GUIDE

ASTHMA &
ALLERGIES

ANN KENT

WITH THE HELP OF THE
NATIONAL ASTHMA CAMPAIGN

WARD LOCK

Ann Kent
Ann Kent is a freelance health writer whose work is published in national newspapers,
magazines and the medical press. She started her career on local and regional
newspapers, and spent seven years as a reporter and feature writer on the Daily Mail
before specializing in health matters. She is currently health editor of Take a Break
magazine, and lives with her teacher husband and four children in Suffolk, England.

A WARD LOCK BOOK

First published in the UK 1994
by Ward Lock
Villiers House
41/47 Strand
London
WC2N 5JE

A Cassell Imprint

Designed and produced
by SP Creative Design
147 Kings Road, Bury St Edmunds, Suffolk, England

Editor: Heather Thomas
Art director: Al Rockall
Designer: Rolando Ugolini
Illustrations: Rolando Ugolini

Distributed in the United States
by Sterling Publishing Co., Inc.
387 Park Avenue South, New York, NY 10016-8810

Distributed in Australia
by Capricorn Link(Australia) Pty Ltd
2/13 Carrington Road, Castle Hill, NSW 2154

A British Library Cataloguing in Publication Data block for this book may be obtained
from the British Library.

ISBN 0 7063 7252 2

Printed and bound in Spain

Acknowledgements
The publishers and author would like to acknowledge the invaluable help given to them
by the National Asthma Campaign in producing this book. Also its medical advisor, Dr
Martyn Partridge for his help in preparing the text.
Cover photograph: Comstock Photo Library
MEDIC-AID: pages 42, 60, 71, 72
National Asthma Campaign: pages 10, 11, 13, 15, 17, 19, 23, 25, 26, 31, 32, 34, 44, 48,
49, 50, 56, 57, 74

Contents

Introduction

Most people with asthma can lead perfectly normal lives, provided that they learn how to control their condition. This type of self management can be very rewarding, but it only works if we are given clear medical advice.

A Mori poll conducted for the National Asthma Campaign in the UK revealed that only one person in fourteen was given 'plenty of information' at the time of diagnosis. Two-thirds of those questioned wanted to know more.

Ann Kent

Yet asthma is not a rare condition, but the most common chronic disease in the Western world. The numbers of people who are affected by it are on the increase, for reasons which are not fully understood.

This book aims to fill the information gap on asthma. It provides a simple explanation of the condition, its causes, the different forms of treatment and the help you can expect to get from your doctor and your local hospital.

Chapter one

The causes of asthma

If you have just been diagnosed as having asthma, you are likely to be shocked and dismayed. The healthy person you used to be before the doctor broke the news has suddenly been turned into a worried patient. If it was your child who was diagnosed, you are now an anxious parent.

In fact, it is sensible to worry a little about asthma, which can still be a life-threatening illness. However, the vast majority of people with asthma live normal lives, and the aim of this book is to show you how to do the same: how to get back to normal.

Asthma affects one child in ten and one adult in 20. Although it claims 2,000 lives a year, the vast majority of people with asthma (3 million in the UK) die from other causes. Nevertheless those 2,000 deaths are particularly tragic because most of them could be avoided. Doctors, friends and relatives who have witnessed a premature and unnecessary asthma death never forget the experience.

As we move towards the twenty first century, life is becoming easier for people with asthma. The early treatments simply dealt with the symptoms of the disease, because little was known about the causes and mechanism of an asthma attack. These days, the newest drugs can often suppress asthma, and, as our understanding improves, it is likely that even more effective treatments will follow.

Intensive research is now aimed at finding the reasons why asthma is on the increase at a time when living conditions have never been more comfortable and disease-free.

The effects of passive smoking, warm but poorly ventilated housing and also traffic emissions are all under suspicion. If the cause or, more likely, causes can be found, then preventionof asthma may actually prove to be the cure.

Asthma is a very individual condition and self-knowledge is an essential part of the treatment. If you or your child has been recently diagnosed with asthma, you do not need to see yourself as a victim of a terrible disease. The challenge you face is to learn all you can about your asthma. You can then use this knowledge to help you avoid those asthma attacks that are avoidable, and to control those that are inevitable.

Remember that most people with asthma are normal, healthy people who lead normal, healthy lives.

The causes of asthma

Asthma – what is it?

Asthma occurs when the airways that supply your lungs with oxygen become narrowed, inflamed, and hypersensitive to your surroundings. When you are exposed to certain triggers, such as tobacco smoke or pollen, the airways tighten, fill with mucus and narrow, and breathing becomes difficult.

Some people have chronic asthma, which means that their breathing is bad all the time, while others have acute asthma attacks, when breathing difficulties occur spasmodically. However, everyone who suffers with asthma has airways which are 'twitchy' and hypersensitive.

We tend to think of our lungs like twin bags which inflate and deflate as we breathe

The respiratory system

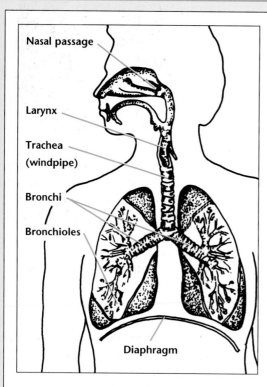

- Nasal passage
- Larynx
- Trachea (windpipe)
- Bronchi
- Bronchioles
- Diaphragm

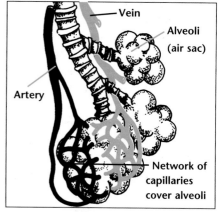

- Vein
- Alveoli (air sac)
- Artery
- Network of capillaries cover alveoli

When you inhale, air enters through your mouth and nose and goes down the windpipe into the lungs through the bronchi(airways). It then enters the smaller airways(bronchioles) and travels into the air spaces(alveoli) where the oxygen is absorbed into the blood, and carbon dioxide is blown out.

in and out. In fact, they are more like sponges. Each lung contains 300 million tiny holes (alveoli) which fill with air as we breathe in, in the same way that a sponge fills with water.

We breathe in and out about 12 times a minute, for most of the time automatically and without effort. When we breathe in, air passes through the nose, into the windpipe and down into two major tubes (the bronchi) which serve each lung.

The bronchi then subdivide a total of 25 times into a network of major and minor airways. The larger airways are supported by cartilage, but the smaller ones lack these supports and are easily compressed as we inhale and exhale.

Air travels along the airways, into the alveoli, and then seeps into the blood circulation. When the air reaches the cells, the oxygen is combined with glucose to release energy.

The waste product of this process of cell respiration, carbon dioxide, is transported through the circulation back to the alveoli. It then passes along the network of airways until it is finally exhaled.

Asthma is a two-stage process. First, your airways become 'twitchy' and in a state where they are constantly inflamed. This inflammation is most likely to be caused by an allergic reaction. However, your airways can also be primed for asthma following a virus infection, or exposure to certain chemicals at work. Once primed, your airways will react in an exaggerated way to triggers that would not bother other people, just as an infected toe will react to the

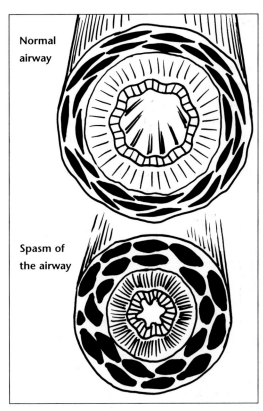

In asthma, the airways narrow and tighten due to inflammation of the linings. Excessive mucus is secreted, the linings swell and the muscles around the airways tighten and go into spasm.

slightest pressure on it.

The second stage occurs when you inhale a substance to which you have become allergic, or a substance which can irritate your airways. This creates further inflammation, tightening of the airways and the simultaneous production of mucus. This is when the symptoms of your asthma – wheezing, coughing and breathing difficulties – really become obvious.

The causes of asthma

Allergic reactions

An allergen is a protein that causes an allergic reaction in susceptible individuals. For instance, you may be allergic to a harmless substance like pollen. When you breathe in the pollen, your body reacts as if you have inhaled a poison. Your immune system will trigger the release of large amounts of the antibody, immunoglobulin E, to destroy the pollen. Unfortunately, this sets off a complex chemical chain reaction which causes the airways to become inflamed and hypersensitive. Although this first reaction will eventually subside, some of the inflammation will remain.

Next time you are exposed to pollen, the same defence mechanisms will be activated,

This photo micrograph shows grass pollen grains which, when inhaled, can be a trigger substance for many asthma sufferers.

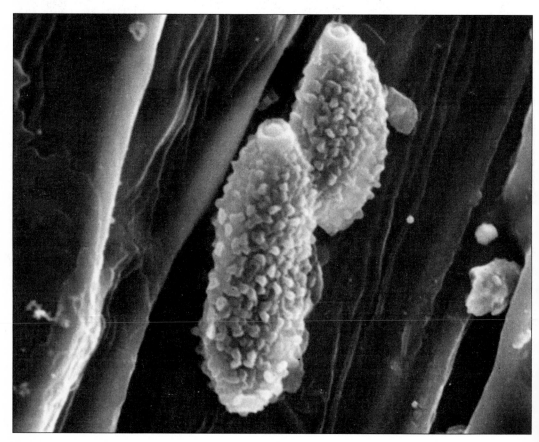

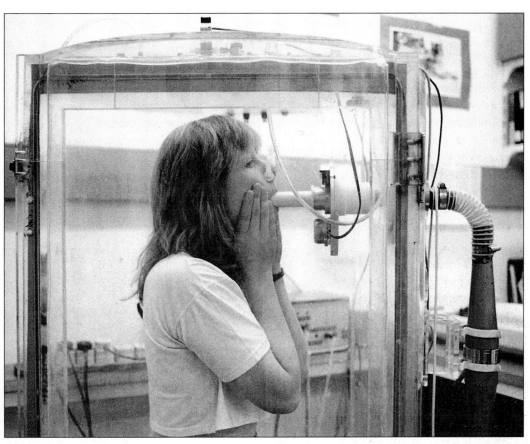

Important research is being carried out into the causes and treatment of asthma by hospitals, medical schools and research institutions all round the world.

and an asthma attack is likely. You are likely to notice symptoms such as wheezing or breathing difficulties when you first breathe in the pollen, and again, several hours later when the chemical chain reaction has had time to work. This means that if you breathe in the pollen in the afternoon, you may suffer asthma symptoms at that time, and then again in the evening or at night. This delayed response is known as a late allergic reaction.

Because the airways are now so hypersensitive, you may now find you also react to a number of other allergens, e.g.

house dust mite, flakes of dog skin and also to irritants which have never really bothered you before, such as cold air, cigarette smoke and aerosol sprays. Substances that provoke your asthma are known as triggers, and vary from one person to the next.

When a trigger substance is inhaled, the airways will respond by constricting and

The causes of asthma

Asthma is rising

There is evidence of an alarming increase in asthma and related allergies, such as eczema and hay fever, over the last twenty years. Doctors and researchers are blaming the rise on a combination of factors: increased air pollution and car exhaust gases, cigarette smoking and passive smoking, home pollutants such as dust mites, and a poor diet with insufficient fresh vegetables and fruit.

In the UK, the number of children suffering from asthma has doubled in a single decade, and now one in ten are thought to be asthmatic. In some cities, air pollution is now reaching levels that can trigger asthma attacks. A UK Parliamentary Office of Science and Technology report, published in 1994, states that the long-term trend in road traffic 'would be consistent with the observed trends in respiratory allergies'. Although, as the report points out, the evidence is not conclusive, vehicle exhaust fumes are the primary cause of pollution.

However, some studies conducted in Britain, Germany and the United States have found little hard evidence of a link between asthma and pollution. Researchers at Aberdeen University medical school in the UK concede that while some air pollutants can damage lung function, poor diet may be a factor too. People in the West are eating less fresh fruit and green vegetables, which are the main sources of vitamin C and beta-carotene, the antioxidant vitamins that boost the immune system. The next step is to investigate whether such a diet has made people more susceptible to respiratory disease, especially asthma.

producing a sticky mucus which further narrows the airways. Breathing, especially breathing out, becomes difficult, leading to a build-up of carbon dioxide in the lungs.

The result may be wheezing, coughing, tightening of the chest or a major asthma attack when the individual is fighting for every painful breath.

An asthma attack is frightening whether you experience it or witness it. It is not surprising that people who are taken unawares by asthma may panic, gulp air, or start to pant.

Trying to relax, adopting the most comfortable breathing pattern possible at this time, and using the reliever inhaler usually helps to bring the attack under control. If the reliever medicine does not work within ten to fifteen minutes then your emergency plan (see page 40) should come into operation. This will always include summoning medical help, or being taken to hospital as soon as possible.

The role of virus infections

Asthma in babies and very young children is usually blamed on virus infections which damage the cells lining the airways, causing them to become hypersensitive and inflamed. Infants often develop asthma after having a series of viral infections, usually 'one cold after another' or flu. However, there is an unresolved 'chicken and egg'! argument about the role of allergy in this type of asthma.

Some scientists believe that babies are particularly susceptible to allergy because their immune systems are poorly developed. They point out that, as a result, the lungs of the babies are particularly susceptible to allergens such as house dust mites, or to irritants such as tobacco smoke. They believe that a virus infection only leads to asthma in babies whose airways were already primed by an allergic reaction. If this turns out to be true, then in future some types of asthma could be avoided by protecting very young children from exposure to allergens, either by adjusting their living conditions, or by vaccination.

However, other researchers believe that it is the damage caused by the virus that primes the baby's airways to over-react to allergens and irritants. At present these arguments do not affect the treatment a child is likely to receive.

Many young children and even babies suffer from asthma. This form of asthma may be caused by viral infections, especially in babies who are susceptible to allergies. Parents of children who wheeze or have a troublesome cough should consult their doctor.

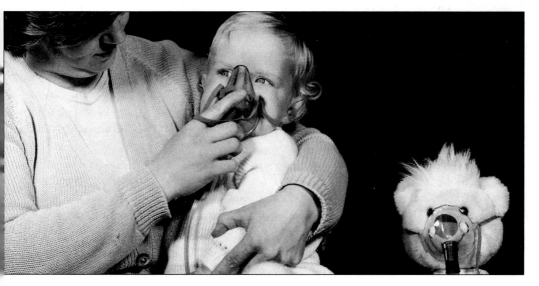

The causes of asthma

Why me? Why my child?

The tendency for people's airways to be hypersensitive is inborn: we inherit this through our genes. Unfortunately, because a combination of genes, rather than a single gene, is involved, it is unlikely that gene therapy will provide an early cure.

We know that asthma tends to run in families that are prone to allergy (atopy). This means that some family members will be affected by asthma, while others may suffer from other allergies such as hay fever, perennial rhinitis (constant inflammation of the lining of the nose) and eczema.

In other words, we inherit a tendency to react to allergens rather than a specific disease. If you or your partner has asthma, there is an increased risk that your children will also be asthmatic, although this is not inevitable.

We tend to think of asthma as being a childhood problem, but it can occur at any age. We may live with our own asthma trigger for years until we suddenly and dramatically develop a sensitivity. Why some people develop asthma so much later than others is not yet known.

Asthma in the over-forties often follows a severe chest infection. In fact, the condition is often misdiagnosed as a return of the infection or a new infection, and it may be some time before the correct treatment is given. Often, some adults who develop asthma late in life report having had a number of chest infections as children.

It is now widely thought that these were probably asthma attacks and that they were mistakenly diagnosed at the time. Asthma can 'go quiet' for many years before flaring up again in later life.

Asthma in families

A tendency to develop allergic asthma and other allergies sometimes runs in a family. Children born to these families are more likely than average to develop asthma, eczema or hay fever. The chances of a child with one asthmatic parent developing asthma are doubled; if both parents are asthmatic, the chances are quadrupled for their children. Allergic parents should try to follow these simple guidelines:

● Try to breastfeed your baby as long as possible(even up to one year), and while you are nursing avoid the foods to which you have been allergic.

● If you are bottlefeeding, it might be a good idea to choose a low-allergy formula.

● Only introduce new foods one at a time, and wait for your child's reaction.

● Do not introduce citrus fruits until nine months.

● Do not offer eggs, cow's milk or wheat until the first birthday.

Talk to your doctor or health visitor about your child's diet, and seek their advice.

What triggers an asthma attack

In many cases people with asthma are sensitive to a number of different allergy-causing substances and irritants. They may not develop an asthma attack until they encounter a combination of triggers, e.g. exercise and cigarette smoke, car exhaust fumes and cold air.

Often, the trigger takes the form of an allergic reaction to a substance which is generally regarded as harmless. Thus, while most people may be able to walk through a newly mown field, an asthmatic who is allergic to grass pollen will start to gasp and wheeze.

If allergic reactions occur in the skin they cause rashes such as eczema, dermatitis and urticaria. When they occur in the eyes and nose (e.g. with hay fever, rhinitis), those organs start to itch and stream. It is not uncommon for people with asthma to have other allergic conditions as well.

The commonest allergic triggers are house dust mites, pollen, animals, mould spores, drugs, chemicals and food. We will examine and explain these in more detail in the following pages.

However, asthma attacks also occur after exposure to a range of non-allergic triggers, including virus infections, exercise, change in temperature, emotional stress, air pollution, hormonal changes (in women) and tobacco smoke.

Many people with asthma have a combination of triggers, allergic and non-allergic. Because of this, doctors are now less inclined to make the distinction between allergic (intrinsic) and non-allergic (extrinsic) forms of asthma.

In the next chapter we will look at triggers and how they can be avoided in more detail.

Inhalers

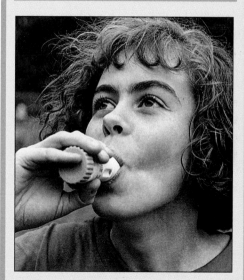

Asthma can be treated by breathing in(inhaling) medicine straight into the lungs. In this way, it can be taken in low doses with minimal side-effects. There are many types of inhalers, including aerosols(puffers), and dry powder devices, which are good for administering preventer treatment to children over three years.

Chapter two

Self-help

If you have asthma, it makes sense to learn as much as possible about your personal triggers. It is no good relying on the knowledge of an asthmatic friend because asthma is a particularly personal condition. Even close relatives with asthma may turn out to have triggers that are quite different from your own ones.

Avoiding asthma altogether would be ideal, but it is seldom possible to banish the condition simply by manipulating your environment. You may have to settle for less, and make changes that will reduce and minimize the number of asthma attacks you have. However, first you need to identify the factors which trigger your asthma.

Allergy testing

There are tests to establish which substances cause an allergic reaction. They involve injecting just a tiny amount of the suspect substance, e.g. house dust mite protein, just under the skin. A reaction occurs when the skin reddens and swells.

However, substances that cause the skin to flare up may not always affect the lungs, so the test result can be misleading. In many cases, people with asthma are able to identify their own triggers by simple observation. If you wheeze whenever a cat walks into the room, you don't need a skin prick test to tell you that you are sensitive to cats. Allergic reactions can also be measured in a blood test to detect the large numbers of antibodies which are released when you encounter an allergen.

However, this test is expensive, and is only used when the exact cause of asthma is proving difficult to pin down.

Testing for food allergy

Sometimes it may be difficult to identify a specific food that is triggering an allergic reaction. Doctors and specialists have four options in diagnosing a food allergy:
● Studying your dietary history: you may have to record everything you eat and how you feel.

● Allergy tests: both skin tests and blood tests are rarely helpful in pinpointing food allergy.
● Challenge tests: these help to ascertain whether a particular food is responsible.
● Exclusion diets: these exclude suspect foods from your daily diet.

16

Finding your trigger

It is likely that you probably have some idea of the triggers that cause your asthma. In an ideal world, you would avoid them all, but often this is impossible. You can shun smoky bars and restaurants, and try to minimize the time you spend outdoors on a frosty day if smoke and cold air are your triggers. However, you cannot lead a normal life while shutting yourself away from the rest of the world, so you will need to compromise.

In fact, even shutting yourself away does not guarantee freedom from asthma attacks. Most people with asthma have a number of triggers, some of which are unavoidable, and some of which they do not even know about.

However, many of these triggers are unmistakeable. You may start to cough and wheeze as soon as you enter a room which is occupied by a dog, or a tight band may wrap itself round your chest when someone sprays an aerosol near your face.

It is important to remember that your breathing difficulties can occur hours after you encountered the irritant.

If you are keen to discover and avoid as many triggers as possible, it is worth keeping an asthma diary. Mark the possible triggers that you encounter from day to day, along with any symptoms you experience. If you are using a peak flow meter, record the readings from this as well.

Typical triggers that would warrant a mention include a walk along a traffic-choked street, a visit to a smoky pub, a trip

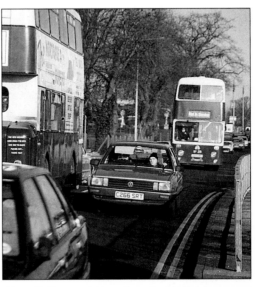

Air pollution and car exhaust emissions can trigger off asthma attacks in some people. Vehicle exhausts produce substantial quantities of nitrogen dioxide which produces low-level ozone in sunlight. This can inflame the bronchial tubes and exacerbate asthma.

to the hairdresser (because of the chemicals and aerosols), temperature changes (e.g. hot and humid, cold and frosty), the effects of a brisk walk across the park (bear in mind that temperature, pollens or exercise could cause symptoms), a cycle ride, or an encounter with a furry animal. You also need to record when you last had a cold, flu or a chest infection.

It is not always possible to identify trigger factors, particularly if your asthma has appeared late in life.

Self-help

Keep a diary

Every day write down the possible triggers that cause your asthma in a diary. Record the peak flow meter readings as well. This will help you not only to pinpoint your personal triggers, but also to avoid them in future so as to minimize asthma attacks.

A typical asthma diary symptoms chart is shown below. You can draw up your own on a sheet of graph paper or use the self-management peak flow charts that are available from your doctor. Recording your symptoms in this way may help you to identify a common pattern and pinpoint your triggers.

Date	Mon	Tue	Wed	Thur	Fri	Sat	Sun	Mon	Tue
Symptoms									
Cough									
Wheeze									
Shortness of breath									

Peak flow	am	pm	am	pm	am	pm	am	pm	am	pm	am	pm	am	pm	am	pm	am	pm
700																		
650																		
600																		
550																		
500																		
450																		
400																		
350																		
300																		
250																		
200																		
150																		
100																		
50																		
0																		

Avoidance

How far you choose to go in avoiding the influences which provoke your asthma is as personal as the condition itself.

Decisions about the family pet are one of the most difficult faced by people with asthma. No one can stop you if you decide to keep the cat, even when it means you need more medication and risk having severe asthma attacks.

The most common allergic trigger to asthma is much less lovable. It is sensitivity to a protein found in the droppings of the house dust mite.

House dust mites

The house dust mite, too small to be seen by the naked eye, thrives on warm, moist conditions. It feeds off the tiny flakes of human skin which we constantly shed as we go about our daily lives.

The richest skin harvest for the mites is to be found in beds and bedding. Even people whose bedrooms are regularly dusted and vacuumed are likely to harbour large numbers of house dust mites.

How the mites should be avoided is controversial. Some authorities recommend a series of measures which have you jumping through hoops, and include the following: washable lino in bedrooms; all bedding washed at high temperatures at least once a week; pillows and duvets with man-made fillings rather than feathers; blinds instead of curtains; no soft toys (or soft toys put in the freezer weekly to kill off mites or washed

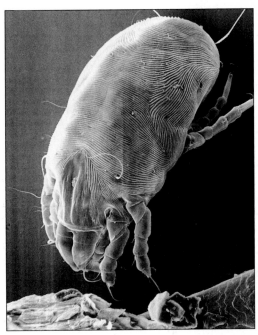

This photograph, which has been magnified 300 times, shows the house dust mite feeding on a human skin cell. Its droppings are the most common allergic trigger to asthma. It predominates in bedrooms, on cushions and carpets – wherever there are human skin scales and warm, humid conditions.

once a week); vacuum cleaners with special filters; insecticide sprays; no central heating; damp dusting; getting someone else to do the housework.

You can try as many or as few of these as you choose; there now seems to be some consensus that damp dusting, and the use of special bedding systems may be helpful.

19

Self-help

Asthma in the home

If you have sensitive airways, there may be trigger factors in your home that can cause wheezing or trigger an asthma attack. However, there are positive measures that you can take to minimize these.

Heating

If your home is damp, you should take steps to eliminate any dampness, which is associated with poor respiratory health.

There is no consensus on which sort of heating is best and least likely to affect or worsen asthma, and very little research has been carried out in this area. Warm houses with central heating are a good breeding ground for the house dust mite, and even when it is cold outside, it is a good idea to leave a window open somewhere and introduce some fresh air into the house. Some people report that ducted air heating causes problems although there is no medical evidence to support this. However, because air is recirculated in this heating system, it is possible that they may breathe in more house dust mite allergen.

People with severe asthma may find that it is affected by gas fire heating with its higher levels of nitrogen dioxide. However, other factors have to be taken into account too, especially passive smoking.

Wood and coal fires with an adequate flue should not cause any problems for asthmatics.

Controlling dust

Dust control is time-consuming but many people report benefits and a gradual improvement in their asthma. Controlled clinical trials have produced varying results, but it might be worth trying the following measures to reduce dust.

● Keep the bedroom dry – house dust mite thrive in warm, damp conditions.

● Wipe flat surfaces, e.g. table tops, window sills, bedside cabinets etc., with a damp cloth every week.

● Replace carpets with vinyl floor covering or linoleum. Add some washable rugs to avoid the problem of cold feet!

● Avoid heavy curtains; use washable light fabrics instead, or roller blinds.

● Shake blankets, pillows, quilts and duvets outside as often as possible.

● Replace feather pillows, eiderdowns, feather-filled duvets and woollen blankets with synthetic ones.

● Use washable plastic covers for mattresses.

● Change all bed-linen once a week.

● Only buy machine-washable soft toys for children, and wash them regularly

● Choose a bed with a plain wooden headboard and frame which collect less dust than beds with upholstered headboards and divan bases.

● If a child is asthmatic, he should sleep in the top bunk.

● Vacuum the mattress at least once a week.

These bedding systems involve impermeable covers for the mattress, pillow, and duvet. You can also buy Slumberland mattresses with mite-proof coverings.

Before you invest in the bedding, you should consider the following: the risk that it may not abolish your asthma (because you have multiple allergies, for instance); the fact that it may take two or three months to notice any results: and the fact that it is not yet known how long the bedding systems remain mite-proof.

You may also be allergic to ordinary house dust. The answer, easier said than done, is to get someone else to do the hoovering, dusting, spring cleaning and turning the mattresses over. Fine wood dust from sawmills can also cause allergic reactions.

Pollen sensitivity

Sensitivity to pollen is also extremely common. The most troublesome plants tend to be wind-pollinated, i.e. grasses, trees and weeds. Tree pollens cause symptoms from April to June, grass pollens from mid May to July, and weeds are pollinated in the spring and the autumn. Allergy to several types of pollen is quite common.

Avoidance involves staying out of long grass, keeping windows closed, especially in mid-morning, and late afternoon or early evening, wearing dark glasses and keeping your car window shut when driving. Many cars have pollen filters, so you may be able to use the cold air blower. If you are planning an outing, check the day's pollen forecast (given on radio, TV and in newspapers).

If you have hay fever as well as asthma,

Tips for avoiding pollen

- Avoid long grass
- Close your windows
- Keep your car windows shut
- Wear dark glasses
- Check the pollen forecast

you can take antihistamines or anti-inflammatory treatments for the nose and eyes. Discuss this with your doctor.

Animals and pets

Animal lovers can find it hard to accept that their pets are a common cause of asthma. Cats and dogs – perhaps because they are kept so often – are the most likely pets to cause trouble. Although animal hair is often blamed because it is visible, flakes of skin (dander) are much more likely to set off allergic reactions. People who are sensitive to horse dander can suffer asthma attacks simply by coming into contact with the clothing of a rider. Furniture and mattresses stuffed with horsehair used to be another common cause of allergy.

In the case of cats, tiny airborne particles of dried saliva often prove to be the allergen. This problem is made worse by the fact that cats are constantly washing themselves. Proteins from the urine of small caged animals, such as mice, hamsters and gerbils, are another common cause of allergy.

Allergy to bird droppings is fairly rare, except among pigeon fanciers who may be heavily exposed to airborne particles when they enter poorly ventilated coops. It is now

al cause of allergy to
and pillows is invasion
, rather than the feathers
themselves.

If you have a strong family history of
allergic problems, or if you or your child is
asthmatic, you should avoid buying a pet.
Even if animals have never been known to
trigger your asthma, sensitization can occur
over a long period. In other words, the
problem may not arise until the cat or dog
has become a much loved family member!

It is worth monitoring asthma symptoms
after visits to friends or relatives with pets to
see if this is making your symptoms worse.
Horse riding, and contact with the clothes of
riders should also be avoided.

But what if a pet is already in residence? If
you are uncertain whether your animal is a
major cause of your problem, go away for a
few days without it (but stay in a pet-free
home). If your asthma seems better, it is worth
repeating the experiment several more times. If
you still seem better, you may want to
consider finding a new home for the animal. If
the asthma is severe, and the sufferer is a child,
the decision may be more clear-cut.

Instant banishment will not provide an

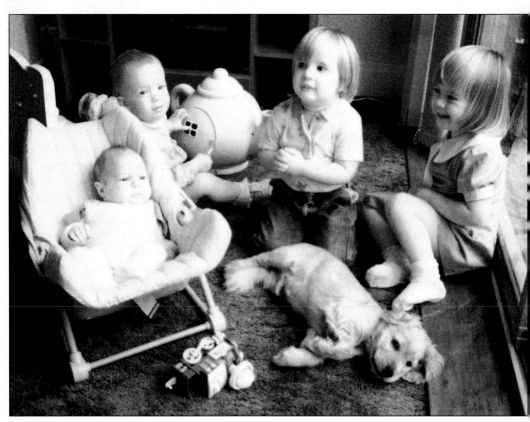

instant answer to your asthma, as the dander can linger in your home for up to three months. Do not expect your asthma to disappear completely even then, because you will still be susceptible to other triggers.

If you are moving house, it is worth enquiring whether your new home has been recently occupied by a pet animal. Some people simply cannot bear to get rid of their pets, and accept that they will need extra medication to coexist with them. How much this matters depends on the severity of the asthma.

Moulds

Another fairly common cause of allergy, moulds are a type of fungi which grow in warm, damp areas and release tiny seed-like particles (spores). They are found on rotting tree trunks in woods, and in damp basements and bathrooms, and even on upholstered furniture in the home.

For many years, doctors have puzzled over why severe asthma attacks often occur after thunderstorms. It has now been found that during a heavy summer storm, large numbers of spores from the mould didymella exitalis, which is found on the leaves of ripening barley and wheat, are released into the air.

Food allergies

The role of food allergy in asthma is still controversial. Some medical experts believe that any attempt to tinker with your diet is likely to be a waste of time. Others accept that asthma can be triggered by food allergy, but emphasise that this is a rare occurrence.

However, many people are convinced

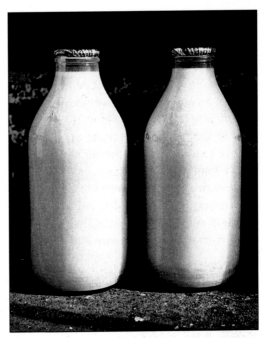

Cow's milk is a common cause of food allergy and may trigger asthma among babies and young children. If you suspect milk, talk to your doctor before excluding it from your child's diet as it is an important source of nutrients.

their asthma is triggered by certain foods, despite what the experts say.

The evidence suggests that some asthma is food-induced. It is likely to occur in people who have multiple allergy symptoms, e.g. eczema or urticaria (nettle rash) as well as asthma. Food-allergic individuals are often sensitive to a number of other allergens as well. For this reason, tracking down the culprit foods may not make much difference to your symptoms.

Identifying food allergy triggers may also be difficult because a late allergic reaction may occur several hours after you have eaten the food (and possibly after you have had another meal). Keeping a symptom diary which includes peak flow measurements may help.

The commonest food allergens are cow's milk (particularly in babies and young children), nuts, soft fruit, shellfish, yeast and yeast products.

Infections

Colds or flu are infections which can often trigger an asthma attack. This is particularly common in babies and young children, but asthmatics of all ages can find that breathing is more difficult, and extra medication is needed, after a viral infection.

Because the infections that cause asthma symptoms are nearly always viral rather than bacterial, they do not respond to antibiotics. If you have just had this kind of illness, you need to be particularly careful about taking your prescribed asthma medication and you may need to increase the dose.

You can't lock yourself away from other people's germs if you are to lead a normal life. However, it may be worth asking your doctor for a flu jab in the autumn to protect you against the commonest type of influenza.

Exercise triggers

Certain types of exercise, particularly running, can cause asthma attacks. In fact, some people's asthma is only caused by exercise. Although tightness in the chest may bring the exercise to an early halt, the worst symptoms of wheezing do not start until a few minutes later. Exercise-induced asthma is more likely at times when your airways are particularly

Warning

It is very easy to be mistaken about children's food reactions, and it is important that you take medical advice before withdrawing important nutrients such as dairy products from their diets.

Food additives can also cause asthma. Research has shown that some people wheeze more if they consume food coloured with the additive tartrazine (E102). These individuals may also react to other dyes, particularly quinoline yellow (E104) and sunset yellow (E110). People who are sensitive to tartrazine or have food allergies are more likely to react to aspirin as well (see aspirin section on page 29.)

Another additive identified as a cause of attacks is sodium metabisulphate. This is an anti-oxidant which is often used in restaurants and in pre-packed foods to keep fruits and salads looking fresh. If you can't drink beer or other fizzy drinks without getting asthma symptoms, it is probably because sodium metabisulphate has been added. It is also used as an ingredient in boxed wines, sausages, meats and some seafood.

irritable, e.g. after you have had a cold, on frosty days or during the pollen season.

Avoiding the exercise trigger altogether is not the answer, especially at a time when more and more research is highlighting the health benefits of keeping fit. Swimming is the ideal sport because the warm, moist air f the pool is least likely to cause symptoms.

Some sportsmen and women with sthma find that a few 30-second sprints just efore vigorous games seems to protect their ungs. Generally, long spells of exercise such s cross-country runs are more likely to nduce asthma than short bursts (e.g. playing occer and cricket).

Pre-treatment helps most people take art in some form of exercise. Compromise is ometimes necessary, such as choosing a less active position in team games rather than avoid playing altogether.

Most people with exercise-induced asthma take a couple of puffs of their reliever inhaler before the exertion begins.

Swimming is the ideal exercise if you have asthma. Breathing in the warm, moist air of an indoor pool rarely causes problems. This girl is competing in a National Asthma Campaign swimming gala in the UK.

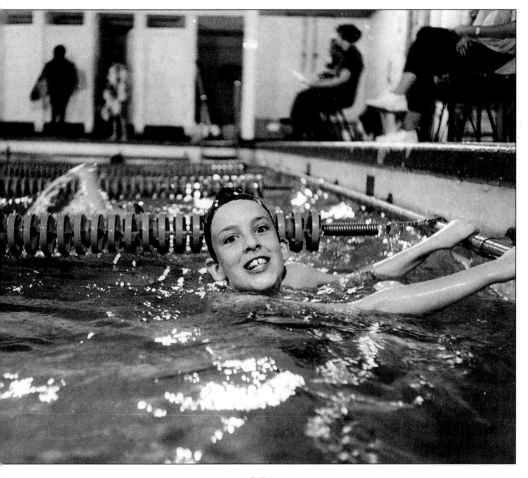

Self-help

Alternatively, they take sodium cromoglycate (a medicine generally used as a preventer which is also effective against exercise-induced asthma) about half an hour before they start to exercise.

If wheezing occurs when the exercise finishes, the reliever inhaler (but not the sodium cromoglycate) can be used again. More detailed information on drug treatments is given later on in the book.

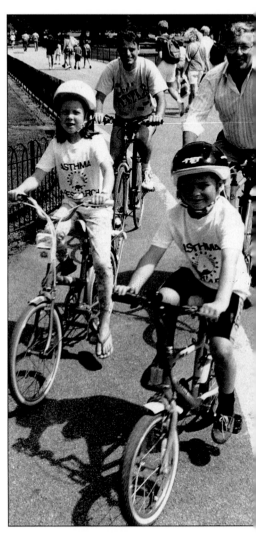

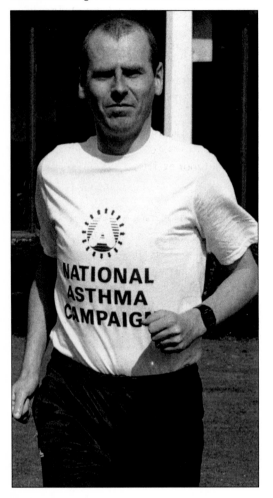

There is no reason why you should not enjoy sports like running and cycling just because you have asthma. Exercise is good for everyone and it is possible to prevent or reduce symptoms by taking medication a few minutes before exercising. Warming up adequately before exercising and abstaining on cold, dry, frosty days may also help.

Air pollutants

Generally, in most Western countries, our air is much cleaner than it used to be. This is certainly the case in the UK when less than 40 years ago the country was sometimes blanketed with thick industrial smogs. Unfortunately, one type of pollution has been replaced by other, less obvious, types.

One of the main causes of air pollution is nitrogen dioxide from motor vehicle emissions. Exhaust fumes have increased by 75 per cent since the 1980s. They are likely to be at their worst when cars are driven for short journeys on cold days, because there are more emissions when the engine is cold.

Although catalytic converters have been fitted to new cars, it is likely to be some time before we see a significant reduction in exhaust fumes.

Nitrogen dioxide has a dual effect in asthma: the toxic fumes irritate the airways and also increase vulnerability to viral infections. Some scientists believe that vehicle exhausts may actually prime the airways of young children for asthma attacks, by making the lungs more sensitive to allergens such as pollen, and more susceptible to damage from viral infections. But this theory, which is supportedby the increase in motor traffic, remains unproven. However, research has revealed a significant link between peak traffic on main roads in Birmingham, and hospital admissions of preschool children with asthma attacks. Further air pollution is caused by pavement level ozone, also known as photochemical smog. This occurs when sunlight reacts with exhaust fumes, and it can inflame the airways of people with asthma and intensify the effects of allergens.

Other air pollutants which make asthma worse include sulphur dioxide, released from power stations, factories and homes when coal is burned; acid air, caused by a reaction of gases such as nitrogen oxide and sulphur dioxide with water vapour; and small pieces of dust or dirt (particulates) blown by the wind or produced when diesel or coal are burned, or from diesel-fuelled motor vehicles.

Air quality gets worse on calm still days when the pollution is not blown away. Poor or very poor air quality is more likely in the winter months.

In most countries air pollution is recorded and may be mentioned on TV and radio weather forecasts. When air quality is poor, you or your children may choose to avoid outdoor exercise.

Smoking

The effects of passive smoking may seem trivial compared to the chemical pollution described above. In fact, inhaling other people's tobacco smoke is the main indoor pollutant and causes a great deal of misery for people with asthma.

Only 15 per cent of the smoke produced by a cigarette is inhaled by the smoker, while the rest is either puffed out or released as sidestream smoke from the cigarette. Passive smoking causes difficulties for nearly six out of ten people with asthma.

Many people who smoke are well aware of the risks to their own health, but they often seem unaware of the hazard they can pose to others. It is reasonable for a person

Self-help

Smoking

Smoking causes 100,000 premature deaths a year in the UK alone, mostly from diseases affecting the lungs and heart. Cigarette smoke contains carbon monoxide and damages the air passages of the lungs, causing them to narrow, and therefore anyone with asthma should not smoke. If you are already a smoker and want to stop this harmful habit, make the decision today to stop now. Motivation is very important if you are to be successful and you should not embark on this course in a half-hearted manner.

If you need help or guidance, ask your doctor for advice on giving up. You may even be able to join a local stop smoking group in your area. Because smoke is an irritant, you will soon notice an improvement, often within 24 hours of giving up.

with asthma to expect to breathe smoke-free air at home, at work, and while enjoying themselves.

In most countries, there are strict laws concerning smoking at work and in public places. Employers may even risk prosecution if someone is harmed because smoking has been allowed in the workplace. If smoky conditions are damaging your health, you should discuss this with your employer.

A growing body of research shows that babies and young children are much more likely to develop asthma if they live in a household which includes smokers. More information on this is given in the section on children and asthma (see page 53).

Smoking when you have asthma involves constantly exposing your airways to a powerful irritant. Most people with asthma find that their condition is variable: the airways are tight on some days, while their breathing is more relaxed and easy on others. In smokers the narrowing can become permanent and hard to reverse, even with treatment. This can lead them to develop two additional conditions, chronic bronchitis and emphysema, which are hard to treat satisfactorily.

Most smokers with asthma improve within 24 hours of giving up. An unlucky minority find that their condition gets worse and the airways become more irritable for a few days. However, this irritability fades, so it is worth persevering.

Millions of people have quit smoking without using any particular method. However, heavy smokers are often hooked on nicotine. If you have tried and failed before, and you really want to give up, it is worth asking your doctor for advice about the latest nicotine replacement therapies, e.g. patches and chewing gum. These treatments should help you deal with your nicotine craving, but they will not remove your urge to smoke in the way that a paracetamol will remove a headache.

Other triggers

Aerosols are best avoided as they can irritate the airways and provoke an attack. In many cases, alternatives now exist.

Emotional stress and even laughing fits (in children) can bring on asthma symptoms. Most of us cannot avoid the unexpected stresses which life brings, and worrying about the effects may make things worse. If you would like to get to grips with your stress, it is worth considering one of the complementary therapies listed in Chapter Six. Some women find their asthma symptoms are influenced by their hormones, particularly in the week before their periods are due. If you suspect this applies to you, check that your symptoms are not being caused because you are taking aspirin or other painkillers. If premenstrual worsening of asthma is very troublesome you need to consult your doctor, as hormonal drugs are sometimes needed.

Some people with asthma are dismayed to discover that changes in the weather can affect them. Cold dry air has an irritant effect which tightens the airways. Exercising in cold air may also increase your symptoms of exercise-induced asthma.

If you know you are going to have asthma symptoms when you step out on a cold day, take a puff of reliever treatment first. You could also cover your mouth and nose with a scarf. Some people's asthma is switched on by other weather changes, including an increase in temperature.

About one person in 20 with asthma finds their condition gets worse after taking aspirin. Sensitivity can develop after years of taking aspirin without problems. In any case, children under the age of 12 should not take aspirin because of the links between the drug and a serious condition known as Reye's syndrome.

Aspirin belongs to a class of drugs known as non-steroidal anti-inflammatories. The painkiller, ibuprofen, and a number of drugs used to treat rheumatoid arthritis also come into this category. If you are buying an over-the-counter painkiller, paracetamol is a better choice.

You should also try to avoid the class of prescribed drugs known as beta-blockers. These are used in tablet form to treat high blood pressure and angina and as eyedrops, in the treatment of glaucoma. Beta-blockers are bad news because they block the effect of adrenaline – a hormone which relaxes the muscles surrounding the airways and makes breathing easier.

Your doctor should be aware of these problems. However, busy doctors and specialists treating you for problems which are not related to asthma can make mistakes. If you are concerned about drugs you are taking for other conditions, always double-check with your doctor that they are safe for you.

Industrial processes

These can expose us to chemical fumes and dusts which can make asthma worse, particularly when glues, paints and plastics are involved. This can create asthma in people who were not previously affected (a condition known as occupational asthma), and also make existing asthma attacks worse. You should look out for the following clues:

Self-help

• Your asthma gets worse during the working week, although symptoms may occur after work, or at night.
• After several days away from work, or on holiday, you notice an improvement.

You can work in a job for months or years before occupational asthma develops. For more information on occupational asthma, see the Useful Information section at the back of this book.

Occupational asthma

The following industries use substances which may provoke occupational asthma. As you will see, these allergens do not just affect a few unlucky individuals involved in obscure manufacturing processes. Very large numbers of people are exposed to them.

1 Platinum refining: platinum salts.
2 Polyurethane foam manufacture, paint spraying (where it involves 2-part polyurethane paints): isocyanates.
3 Paint manufacture, processes using 2-part epoxy resin paints and adhesives: epoxy resin curing agents and hardening agents including phthalic anhydride, tetrachlorophtalic anhydride, trimellitic anhydride or triethylenetetramine.
4 Electronics industry: colophony fumes arising from the use of rosin as a soldering flux.
5 Detergent industry: proteolytic enzymes
6 Milling, baking farming: dusts arising from sowing, cultivation, harvesting, drying, handling, milling, transport or storage of barley, oats, rye, wheat or maize; or the handling, transport or storage of flour made from them.
7 Textile manufacture: reactive dyes.

8 Carpentry, joinery, papermilling, sawmilling: wood dusts, e.g. cedar and mahogany.
9 Manufacture and administration (e.g. nurses): isphagula dust (a component of bulk laxatives).
10 Merchant navy, laboratories, felt making: castor bean dust.
11 Preparation of ipecacuanha tablets: ipecacuanha.
12 Expanded foam plastic manufacture: the blowing agent azodicarbonamide.
13 Hospitals, histology, electron microscopy, leather tanning, cooling towers: glutaraldehyde.
14 Hairdressing: persulphate salts and henna.
15 Laboratories, pest control, fruit cultivation: insects, other anthropods and their larvae.
16 Food processing: crustaceans or fish or their products, soya bean, tea dust, green coffee dust.
17 Drug manufacture: antibiotics, cimetidine
18 Welding: fumes from the welding of stainless steel.

Chapter three

Taking control of your asthma

Taking control of your asthma is the best way of getting back to normal. But control goes much further than avoiding the triggers that set off an attack.

Although your doctor will have prescribed some medication, you will take charge of how it is used. Unless you have a personal physician in constant attendance, you will have to make some treatment decisions when your symptoms get bad – decisions such as whether to ring for help, make an appointment to see your doctor, or otherwise go straight to the hospital.

Your doctor has no way of knowing when your medicine is failing in its job, so it is up to you to seek out medical help.

No one likes to have to carry medicines around with them. It underlines the fact that you are 'different' and one way of denying illness is to constantly forget to pack your puffer. However a couple of discreet puffs of the inhaler is much less likely to emphasise your difference than a distressing asthma attack in public.

Drug treatments

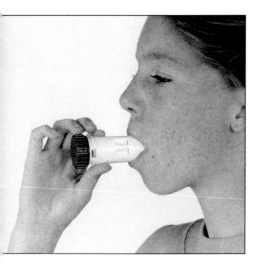

Until the l980s, asthma treatments relied heavily on bronchodilators. These ease breathing by relaxing the muscles which surround the airways.

Bronchodilators are still used to relieve asthma symptoms as they arise. However, these reliever drugs do nothing to reduce the inflammation which makes the airways hypersensitive to triggers. For this reason nearly everyone with asthma is now also given preventive treatments to damp down the inflammation.

In children, sodium cromoglycate (Intal) is often used as a preventive treatment.

Taking control of your asthma

Adults use low doses of inhaled steroids such as beclomethasone (Becotide or Becloforte) or budesonide (Pulmicort) or fluticasone (Flixotide).

Most asthma drugs are designed to be breathed in, so they can work directly in the airways. This allows smaller doses to be used than when drugs are taken in tablet form.

The inhaled drugs are delivered by means of aerosols (puffers), dry powder inhalers, spacers and nebulisers (see page 65).

Sometimes it is necessary to take both preventive and reliever medicines in tablet form. More information about the different drugs prescribed for asthma and their side effects is given in Chapter Five.

Peak flow meters

The peak flow meter records the speed at which air can be blown out of the lungs. The narrower the airways, the more difficult it becomes to force out the air, and the lower the reading. In people who do not have asthma, the variation between readings is never more than 15 per cent. If you have asthma, the difference between readings will be much greater. Doctors often ask patients to take readings on waking (when the reading is likely to be low), in mid afternoon (when it reaches a high) and just before bed (low again).

Peak flow meters can help you monitor your condition, identify asthma triggers, warn of asthma attacks, show when your medication is working, and help assess the severity of an asthma attack. In cases of doubt, they help doctors decide whether or not an individual is suffering from asthma (although other symptoms are also taken into account).

They are most likely to be needed when asthma is moderate or severe, and in the UK are available on prescripton. They will help keep your asthma under control.

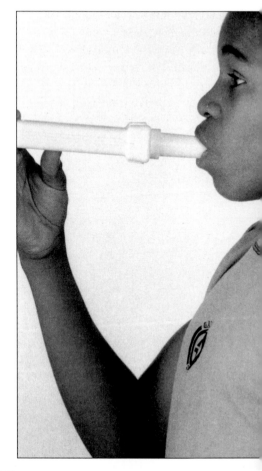

Measuring peak flow

Peak flow charts are a useful indicator of the health of your lungs and how well your treatment is working. They are a way of diagnosing asthma and may help to identify what is triggering your asthma. Measuring your peak flow scores before and after treatment may help to reveal the effectiveness of the medication being used. They are also useful in preventing asthma attacks, as regular readings can give you early warning of a forthcoming attack and you can increase your treatment to help avoid them.

A sign that your asthma may be getting worse is if your scores often fall below your normal. Another tell-tale clue is bigger differences between scores taken in the mornings and evenings. Testing your own asthma in this way is an important part of devising your own self-management plan and bringing it under control. See page 35 for further information on this.

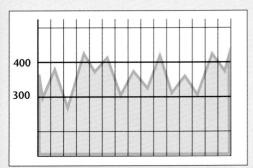

Up and down scores may point to asthma.

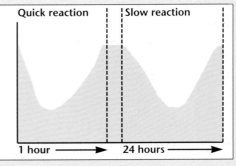

Scores may show a quick reaction to some factors and a slower one to others.

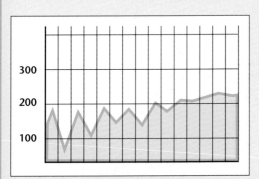

Medicines are working more effectively when scores even out and are less up and down.

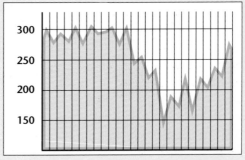

A drop in score is an advance warning of an attack.

Taking control of your asthma

What to expect from your doctor

One of the best ways of regaining control of your health is to ensure that your asthma treatment is the best that is available. So how do you achieve this?

The Asthma Manifesto, published by the National Asthma Campaign in the UK, states that people with asthma have the right to:

- Select the best inhaler device for them.
- Monitor their own condition using a peak flow meter.
- Control their asthma by following an agreed self-management plan.

Asthma specialists meet regularly at conferences where they share their findings and set common standards for the best treatment of patients. These meetings have resulted in a number of recent changes in the way asthma is managed.

There is a new emphasis on long-term

> ### The asthma manifesto
>
> This states that if you have asthma you have certain rights, including the following:
> **1** You have the right to select the best inhaler device for you.
> **2** You have the right to monitor your own condition, using a peak flow meter.
> **3** You have the right to control your asthma by following an agreed management plan.

preventive treatments, with the reliever treatments taking secondary importance.

The complete control of asthma with preventive treatments means that the relievers may hardly need to be used at all.

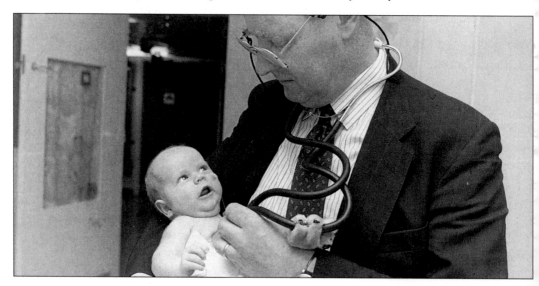

Family doctors

Patients should expect their doctors to be up to date, and to follow these agreed policies. According to the British National Asthma Campaign's manifesto, trained professionals should review the way an individual's asthma is managed at least once a year. Often, doctors or asthma nurses will want to do this even more often.

In the UK, your treatment may be shared between your doctor and the practice nurse. If this is the case, the practice nurse should have received specialist training.

Individual doctors have very different styles. Some 'caring, sharing' types discuss everything with you, while others take a more paternalistic approach and expect you to expect them to be doing their best.

It may be that doctors in this second group are just as up-to-date as the 'caring, sharing' ones. The only way you can find out

is by asking them questions about what measures you can take to prevent asthma attacks. Your doctor should also be able to help you to identify possible triggers.

In the UK, family doctors are given extra payments for setting up asthma clinics – special sessions where all their patients have asthma. Nevertheless, if your doctor runs a clinic the chances are that he or she has a special interest and expertise in asthma.

If your doctor is not interested in your condition, you can now sign on with a new family doctor, without having to give an explanation to your old one, provided that the new doctor agrees to take you on. If you want to find a doctor with a special interest in asthma and you live in the UK, you could ask your nearest National Asthma Campaign branch whether they know of one locally (see page 79 for details).

Self-management plans

It is very useful to agree a self-management plan with your own doctor. This gives specific, detailed information which is personal to you about how to cope with your asthma.

The plan, which should be written down, may be based partly on peak flow readings. For instance, if your peak flow falls below a certain level, the management plan will recommend extra reliever medicine. If it falls lower still, the plan may suggest that you start a short course of steroid tablets.

Research has shown that people who follow such plans end up taking less medication.

However, no matter how foolproof your plan seems to be, it is not intended as a substitute for your own doctor.

If your asthma starts to get worse (or much better) you should tell your doctor immediately so that he or she can make any necessary changes to your medication.

It is tempting to soldier on without bothering the doctor – apart from the

Taking control of your asthma

occasional repeat prescription. In fact, you have a better chance of keeping your asthma under control if you tell your doctor about any day-to-day changes in the nature or frequency of your asthma attacks.

However not everyone will want the responsibility of a self-management plan. Even if you prefer to leave this kind of fine tuning to your doctor, it is important to discuss with him what you should do when you have an asthma attack, and how to act in an emergency. This information should be given verbally, and also in writing so it is also available to people who may be caring for you.

You will find that more information on what to do in an emergency and how to handle it is given later in this chapter.

Controlling your asthma

There are positive steps that you can take yourself to control your asthma on a day-to-day basis. To help you manage your asthma, doctors have devised a 'stepwise treatment plan'. This consists of a series of steps which relate to treatment. If you find that the treatment for one step is not keeping your asthma under control, then your doctor will probably advise you to move up to the next step. However, if your asthma is under control, then he may recommend that you move down a step and decrease the treatment you are taking.

For this treatment plan to be effective, you must be in regular contact with your doctor and report to him on your progress. He can then decide whether to increase or decrease your medication. Below are the five steps to managing adult asthma. Note that this plan relies on teamwork between you and your doctor – you should not attempt it on your own.

Step 1

Your asthma is under control and you sometimes use a short-acting reliever. However, if you are using it more than once daily, your doctor may recommend that you go up one step.

Step 2

You need to take regular preventer treatment to reduce inflammation in your airways, perhaps a steroid inhaler, as well as your short-acting reliever.

Step 3

You need to take higher doses of regular preventer treatment or long-acting relievers, as well as your short-acting reliever. You may also now need to use a spacer.

Step 4

As well as your short-acting reliever and high-dose preventer treatments, you may also need to take a long-acting reliever and/or a different type of short-acting reliever.

Step 5

In addition to your other treatments, you may also be given single daily doses of steroid tablets.

Hospital doctors

The National Asthma Campaign manifesto states that people with asthma have the right to expect to be seen by a specialist whenever necessary. For adults, the specialist is usually a consultant in respiratory medicine.

Consultants work in teams, with senior registrars, registrars and senior house officers. Although any of these doctors may see you in the outpatients clinic, they work under the authority of the consultant.

Children should be seen by a consultant paediatrician with a special interest and expertise in asthma treatment.

If you and your doctor are together controlling your asthma, then referral to a specialist may not be necessary. If you feel it is necessary, you can ask your doctor to refer you, but you have no legal right to insist on this. Talk to your doctor about any worries that you might have.

Emergency treatment

The NAC manifesto also states that in an emergency, you have the right to expect your call for help to be treated as urgent by all health professionals, especially doctors, practice nurses and receptionists. In fact, health professionals do usually take asthma attacks very seriously indeed.

You also have the right to expect a swift response by an ambulance staffed with

trained paramedics, and equipped with both oxygen and nebulisers. On arrival in the accident and emergency department, you should be given priority as an urgent case.

If these standards are not met and you live in the UK, then your local community health council (listed under this title in the phone book) can advise you on how to complain about your treatment.

Coping with an asthma attack

Dealing with an asthma attack competently is one way of keeping your life as normal as possible. If the attack is severe, other people may need to do the coping for you. It is well worth talking to friends and relatives about what might happen and how they can help you if you do suffer a bad attack and cannot cope on your own. They can help you use

your medication, work the nebuliser, or ask you if you need a doctor or ambulance. Even if you can't speak you can usually nod or shake your head to communicate your wishes to them. Explain to them about your asthma and the drugs you take. Show them how to use a nebuliser so that they are well prepared and know what to do in the event of a bad attack.

Taking control of your asthma

How to treat an asthma attack

You will probably recognise the warning signs that your asthma is slipping out of control and that you may be going to have an asthma attack. You can take the normal preventive measures, but if you do have an attack, you need to know how to cope and what action you should take.

Action plan

1 Take a high dose of your reliever medicine. If it is not solving your breathing difficulties, then try the reliever again after five to ten minutes. During this time, it is very important to try and stay calm, and to relax as much as your breathing will allow you to do so.
2 Don't lie down; sit in a position that feels comfortable to you. If you like, you can lean forwards, keeping your back straight, and rest your arms on a table or any firm surface. Alternatively, rest your hands on your knees to help support your back.
3 Loosen any tight clothing around the neck, e.g. a neck tie or top buttons on a shirt. If it very warm, open a window and let in some fresh air.
4 Reliever medicines usually work quickly and if there is no improvement within 15 minutes you should contact your doctor or local hospital immediately.

Important

You should never delay seeking medical help. If your reliever is not working, you must call the doctor or an ambulance. Do not worry about causing a fuss or being a nuisance. If your doctor is contacted in time, he might be able to administer some medication that will deal with the attack.

First aid

If you are with someone who is having an asthma attack, follow the general guidelines set out above. Do not panic; stay calm and try to reassure the person having the attack. Encourage him to breathe slowly and deeply. Assist him with taking any prescribed medicines, e.g. inhalers, nebulisers etc. Find out what sort of reliever medicine he has. If he has only an inhaler, it may help to make an emergency spacer device with a disposable plastic, paper or polystyrene coffee cup(see page 69). If he shows no improvement within 15 minutes, despite taking medication, you must ring the doctor or emergency services. Continue with the reliever treatment until medical help arrives. If he has any of the following severe symptoms, you should seek medical advice immediately.

- If he starts to go blue around the lips.
- If he becomes confused, drowsy or exhausted by the attack.
- If he has really severe diffuculties in breathing.
- If he finds it difficult to speak.

Warning signs

Asthma attacks can occur very suddenly. As you get used to having asthma you may notice very personal symptoms such as an itchy feeling in the skin or nose, light-headedness, nausea, or a tickly cough. Children, in particular, are likely to notice that their skin itches in the top part of their bodies. It may be possible to avoid an attack by taking extra medication at this time.

Other warning signs that your asthma could run out of control include the following:
● Changes in your peak flow meter recordings including: falling readings; morning dips; and increased gaps between the morning and evening readings.
● A more frequent need for reliever medicines, or the discovery that they don't seem to open the airways as well as usual.

● Waking up at night with coughing, wheezing, shortness of breath or chest tightness.
● Your usual symptoms of asthma seem to get worse.
● Inability to maintain your usual activities and exertions.

Ideally, the asthma management plan you have discussed with your doctor should include advice about how to handle warning signs. If you have any of the above signs you should discuss the situation with your family doctor as soon as possible. Follow his or her advice.

If you have received no advice, it is worth taking extra puffs of your reliever medicine. If this does not help within 20 minutes, then you must seek urgent medical attention.

reating an asthma attack

your reliever medicine is not helping after ve to ten minutes (or you have no access to , you may have an asthma attack. Most thma attacks can be managed in the home, ithout the need for hospital admission. his is the time when any efforts you have ade to educate friends and relatives about w to act should bear fruit. You should:
Keep trying the reliever.
Try to stay calm and relax (easier said than ne, but it does help).

● Sit in a position which you find comfortable, and resist attempts to lie you down as this restricts your breathing.
● Some people find it helps to sit leaning forward, with hands resting on knees.
● Try to slow your breathing down.

Treating a bad attack
Your asthma management plan should also include how to treat a bad attack, where admission to hospital may be necessary.

Taking control of your asthma

If you have the following warning signs, then you need to call your family doctor immediately. If the doctor is not available, you should call for an ambulance (or have someone call one for you), or arrange to be driven to hospital. The signs are that:

● You are unable to complete sentences without gasping for breath.

● Your asthma is not responding to the extra doses of reliever medicines.

● Breathing continues to be very difficult.

● Your lips or tongue go blue.

● Your pulse and breathing are very fast.

● You are exhausted.

Once you are sure help is on the way, you can take 15 to 30 puffs of your reliever medication. If you have been given steroid tablets to cover this contingency, then take them if you can.

Asthma attacks are always unnerving, but people with severe asthma say that they do become less frightened of bad attacks in time and are better able to cope with them when they happen.

If your asthma is out of control, do not hesitate to cause a fuss. Inability to breathe a medical emergency and a threat to your life. This is no time to be polite.

What happens in hospital

If you are rushed to hospital, it helps if you can remember to take all of your asthma medications with you. Doctors will want to know what steroids you have taken, whether a nebuliser has been used, and if you are already taking the drug theophylline, because giving more of this drug can be dangerous.

When you arrive in the accident and emergency department the doctor will examine your chest and check your pulse, blood pressure, and peak flow. A blood test may also be taken to check oxygen and carbon dioxide levels in the blood, or, alternatively,

the oxygen level may be measured by a simple probe which is placed on the finger.

Your treatment usually begins with a nebuliser, which should slightly improve the peak flow reading. If you need to be admitted to hospital, a chest X-ray may be taken to check that no damage to the lungs has occurred during the asthma attack.

On the ward, you are likely to be given regular nebulised bronchodilator treatment and steroid injections. Oxygen may also be needed, and in the most severe cases, you could need a ventilator. As you improve, the treatments are gradually reduced.

Chapter four

Children, allergy and asthma

Most primary school classrooms contain one or two children with asthma. One child in ten is affected by the condition, although many grow out of it by the time they reach adolescence. However, their asthma may return, for unknown reasons, at some later stage in their lives.

Symptoms which suggest a child has asthma include the following:

● Repeated attacks of wheezing and coughing, usually with colds.

● A cough which won't go away or keeps coming back, and which may be particularly noticeable at night.

● Restless nights due to wheezing or coughing.

● Wheezing and/or coughing between colds, especially after exercise, excitement, exposure to cigarette smoke and allergic triggers such as dust, pets and pollens.

● Children who get colds which go on to the chest and take more than two weeks to get better.

For many young children, a dry irritating cough can be the only symptom of asthma. Coughs are sometimes dismissed too lightly by doctors and parents; healthy children do not have a perpetual cough.

The hypersensitive airways of asthmatic babies and toddlers appear to be triggered by a chest infection, and scientists are still researching whether allergy may have a 'priming' effect in this process. In older children, their asthma is usually caused by an allergy, or more usually by a series of different allergies.

It is quite common for allergy testing to show that children are sensitive to all the common allergic triggers.

Luckily, sensitivity to one particular trigger is not always enough to set off an asthma attack. However, if that trigger is combined with other allergens and irritants, e.g. pollen plus pets plus someone else's tobacco smoke, an attack may occur. For this reason, it is always worth trying to reduce your child's exposure to allergens even if you cannot banish them all.

Try keeping a diary which records your child's symptoms and any possible allergens he or she has encountered, and show it to your doctor. Even if you suspect food allergy, see the warning in the food allergy section on page 24. People who are allergic to certain specific foods also tend to have multiple allergies.

Children, allergy and asthma

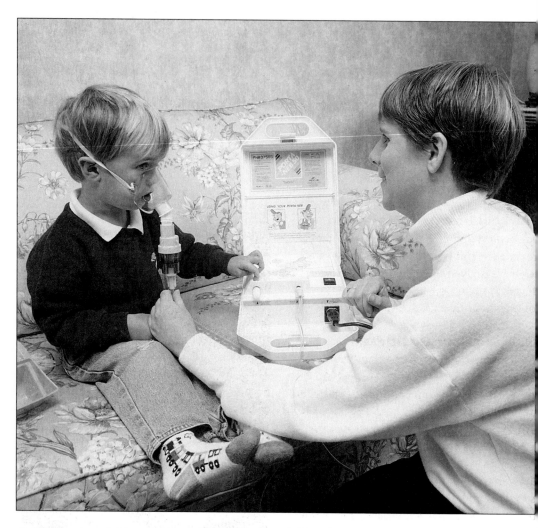

Asthma and the under fives

Three preschool children in ten develop a wheeze, but for many youngsters this is a one-off occurrence and does not necessarily turn into asthma.

Diagnosing asthma can be difficult in young children because they are unable to use peak flow meters, and find it difficult to

Using a home nebuliser is very simple and may be recommended by your doctor or prescribed by your hospital consultant if a child needs extra help to take his medication. The nebuliser creates a mist of medicine for the child to inhale.

describe their symptoms accurately to you.

Sometimes, doctors resolve their doubts by testing whether the child's

mptoms get better with the use of an
.thma treatment such as salbutamol
/entolin) syrup.

Asthma is unusual below the age of one
ear, possibly because it takes time for the
rways to become sensitized to irritants and
llergic triggers. When it does happen in
babies, it often starts after a viral infection,
e.g. flu, measles, or a series of colds.

Bronchiolitis, an infection of the
smallest airways inside the lungs, can often
lead to asthma. Babies who have already had
eczema or colic also seem to be at greater risk
of developing the condition.

Treatment

etailed information about different asthma
eatments, and the way in which they are
elivered is given in the following chapter.
lowever, there are also some special
onsiderations to take into account.

reating young children

etting medicines into babies and young
hildren with asthma can be difficult. An
ngry, off-colour toddler is likely to spit out
iedicines in syrup form, is unable to use an
rdinary inhaler (puffer) and may struggle
nd fight against a face mask.

Dealing with these problems for the first
me can be nearly as distressing for the parent
s for the child. However, even a child who is
truggling and crying will inhale some asthma
iedication. Do not hesitate to ask your doctor
r asthma nurse to show you the best way to
o this and to give you some general advice
n how to cope with these problems. Until
ecently, nebulisers were the most popular way
f giving medicines to children who were too
oung to manage inhalers. Now spacer
evices, which are more portable and simpler
o use, are gaining in popularity.

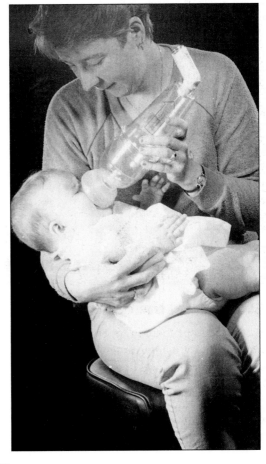

Children, allergy and asthma

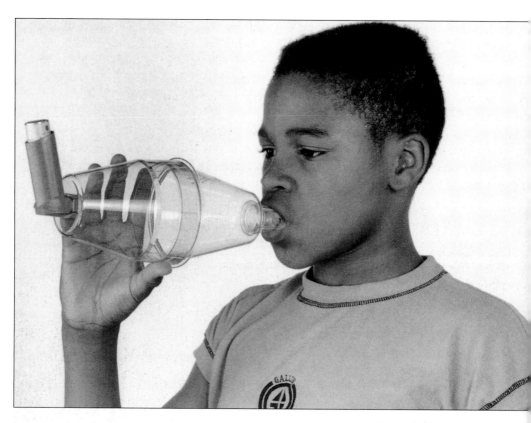

Spacers

Spacers (apart from the new Aerochamber) usually come in two clear plastic halves, which click together to form a chamber. When the device is assembled, it has a mask for the child at one end and a hole for the inhaler at the other. The parent then squirts the aerosol into the spacer, one puff at a time, allowing the child to take five to ten breaths between puffs. The child breathes through the spacer mask, inhaling the drug from the chamber.

Spacers deliver the aerosol with less force than a standard puffer, so that the drug is

Spacers are more efficient than inhalers alone and get the medicines into the child's lungs effectively and safely. They are particularly good for giving inhaled medicines to small children for whom just an inhaler is no good.

less likely to be deposited at the back of the throat and swallowed. Unlike the standard aerosols, the child does not have to co-ordinate breathing in with the activation of the aerosol.

If the spacer is forgotten, an emergency spacer can be made by making a hole in the base of a paper cup for the puffer. The wide nd of the cup is placed over the child's nose nd mouth, and the aerosol is activated.

If your baby will not tolerate anything eld against the mouth, you can hold the ask near and just below the face. However, ou may need to tip the spacer to keep the alve open. The infant will still breathe in e medication, even though some is lost.

You may need a lot of reassurance while ou are learning to deal with your child's

asthma. Your doctor will understand how worrying it can be to try to get medication into a wheezing child, and should not object to being contacted out-of-hours if you are experiencing problems with this.

Nebulisers

If you have a nebuliser, keep it in a special place, and make sure that all the parts are there, ready to be set up, and you always

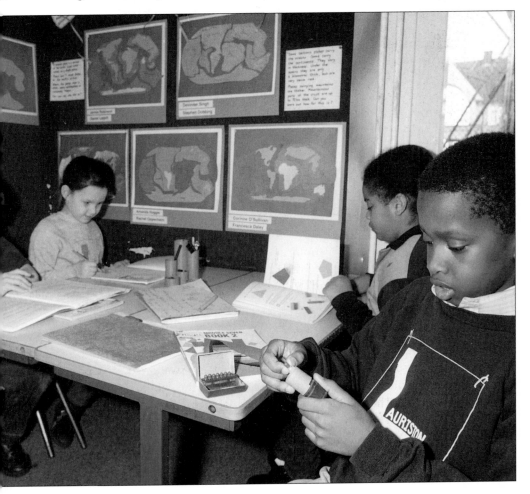

Children, allergy and asthma

have a stock of nebuliser solution handy.

Nebulisers deliver higher doses of drugs than do aerosols. You should talk to your doctor about whether your child would benefit from a home nebuliser before making the decision to buy one because spacers are cheaper, and often equally effective.

Treating older children

Treating asthma in slightly older children is simpler because standard inhalers can be used. These can be slipped easily into a pocket or school bag, and are thus easier to carry (but also, possibly, easier to forget).

From the age of six, children can use peak flow meters which makes it easier to monitor changes in their condition. They also help check how well treatments are working.

Children who are old enough to ask you questions deserve a simple explanation of their asthma. Always use the word 'asthma' rather than evasive phrases like 'weak chest' or 'bad cold'. In the UK, the National Asthma Campaign runs a Junior Asthma Club for children under 12 who have asthma. The address is at the back of this book.

When treatment seems to fail

In addition to the warning signs discussed in the previous chapter, your child may have a personal signal, e.g. an irritating dry cough, or an itchiness of the skin.

How you respond to these warning signs depends on the strategy you have agreed with your doctor. If your child's symptoms increase, or your child needs more reliever medicine, you should inform your doctor

Spotting asthma

Patterns to look for include:
● Repeated attacks of wheezing and coughing, often with colds.
● A persistent cough, which doesn't seem to go away.
● Wheezing and/or coughing when the child doesn't have a cold, e.g. after exercise, when excited, when exposed to cigarette smoke or dust, pets, pollen, feathers etc.
● Waking at night, wheezing and/or coughing.

immediately. It is possible that more of the preventive treatment is needed.

However, more drugs are not always the answer when treatment seems to be failing. Your child may not be using the inhalers properly. Children often try to rush through their treatments and sometimes breathe the drug out before they have had a chance to absorb it into their lungs.

Explain this problem to your child, and watch while the treatment is being taken. If you are uncertain as to whether your child is getting it right, ask your doctor or asthma clinic nurse to check.

Treatment may also fail when children are exposed to more irritants and allergens than usual, e.g. a build-up of house dust mites, other people's smoke or a pet in the house. In addition if you are tense and have any worries you may unwittingly be sharing them with your child, and stress can make asthma worse.

46

Treating an asthma attack

Your child will not want to eat, but he will benefit from extra drinks. Talk to your child in a calm reassuring way, and encourage him or her to breathe slowly.

If children have been taught any special breathing exercises, this is the time to use them. Diversions, such as listening to a story or a story tape, watching TV, or doing a puzzle, will take your child's mind off what is happening and will give the treatment time to work.

Treatments will depend on the plan agreed with your doctor (see page 35). Your child may need to take the reliever treatments by nebuliser. Your doctor may bring the equipment round, or you may have one in the house. However, treatment with a spacer device can often be as effective. Nebulisers and spacers are explained in the next chapter. Turn to page 66 for more information.

Don't wake your child if, after treatment, he or she falls asleep and starts to wheeze. Wheezing usually gets louder during sleep.

Treating an uncontrolled asthma attack

Sometimes, despite your best efforts, the asthma does not respond to the treatment you can provide at home. An asthma attack can take anything from a few hours to a few days to develop until the child becomes breathless, and may be unable to feed or talk. how you behave in these conditions is very important. Here are some general guidelines for you to follow:

● Staying calm is essential, even if it means you have to give an Oscar-winning performance. Children are very sensitive to your fear and anxiety.

● Call your doctor or an ambulance or take your child to hospital (whichever is the quickest way of getting expert help).

● If your child is able to swallow them, give the dose of steroid tablets agreed with your doctor for this contingency.

● If the attack is very severe, i.e. the child is going blue and is unable to talk, call an emergency ambulance because extra oxygen will be needed for the journey.

● Give an extra dose of reliever spray before leaving the house, whether you are travelling by car or ambulance.

● If you go to hospital, make sure you take all your child's medications with you to show the doctor.

Once the crisis is past, make sure you have a follow up appointment with the hospital doctor, or your own family doctor. It is worth discussing with the hospital doctor, your doctor (or both), whether your child's hospital admission could have been avoided. You may also need to restock on your child's drugs, including the special solutions needed for the nebuliser.

Children, allergy and asthma

Asthma management plans

It is much easier to stay calm if you know what you are doing, and an agreed treatment plan with your doctor is essential. This will inform you how to react to your child's symptoms, e.g. when you should increase the medication, when to call for medical assistance, and when to go straight to the hospital (or summon an ambulance).

Anxiety can make the mind go blank, and the plan should be written down even if you have a good memory. If you do not have a treatment plan, or you have forgotten the answers, see your doctor as soon as possible. If nothing is provided in writing, be prepared to make notes. In the UK , the National Asthma Campaign publishes a free booklet on self-management plans with a section where the general practitioner or nurse can fill in details of your plan.

If your doctor is not interested enough to provide this information, it is in your child's interest to be registered with one who is and if this is the case you should seriously consider changing your doctor.

In general terms, a management plan for babies might suggest that when symptoms get worse, a dose of reliever medicine is

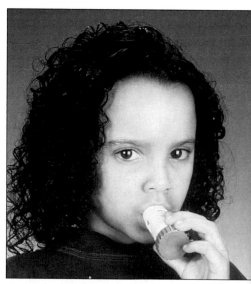

given by plastic cup, spacer, or nebuliser.

The exact details of the plan need to be worked out with your doctor, to ensure it meets the baby's individual needs. You should always report back to your doctor when you have needed to give your child extra medication.

With an older child, the dose of the preventive medicine is increased at the first sign that asthma is worsening. As this will not lead to an immediate improvement, a reliever inhaler is also used.

If the asthma does not respond or peak flow (if measured) continues to fall, the next stage is to give the reliever treatments by nebuliser or spacer at set intervals (often three hourly) until an improvement is seen. Steroid tablets will also be needed for a few days, to damp down the inflamed airways.

Making a plan

Develop an asthma management plan with your doctor which explains when to use the medications and what to do if your child's symptoms get worse.

Asthma at school

Getting back to normal life is particularly important for children, who usually hate to be 'different' and want to be just like their friends, particularly at school.

You need to talk to your child's teacher and possibly the headteacher and explain why it is essential for your child to have access to his or her inhalers. Taking a couple of puffs before exercise is far better than being 'off games' or, worse, being sent home.

Sometimes asthma inhalers are used as playthings by younger children. Spraying asthma medications around is wasteful, but you can reassure the school staff that this will not harm non-asthmatic children. Often the problem can be solved by switching the child to a dry powder inhaler, which seems to be less exciting than an aerosol.

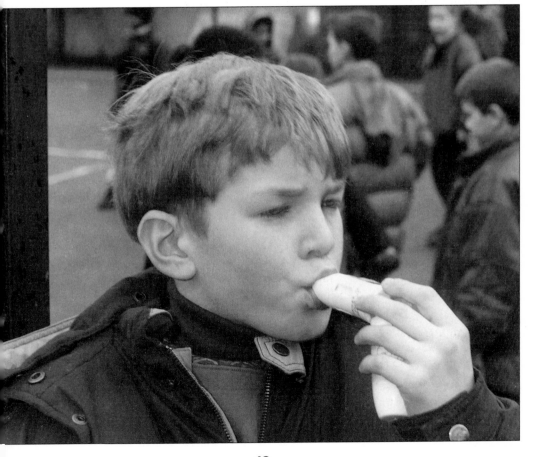

Children, allergy and asthma

Teachers exist to get the best from your children, and they can only do this if your child is as healthy as possible. If you run into difficulties at the school, and they will not co-operate in helping to manage your child's asthma or allowing access to inhalers, perhaps because of a policy which keeps medicines locked away, you may need to start campaigning.

Talk to the chairman of the school governors, and then be prepared to get on to the local education office. In the UK, the National Asthma Campaign has a school policy which can be adapted for your school and includes helpful advice and information for head teachers and members of a school's teaching staff.

Your peak flow meter should help you assess when a child is fit enough to go to school. Unless your child is mixing noxious substances in the chemistry laboratory, or caring for the class hamster, he or she is likely to encounter fewer allergens in the classroom than at home.

Children, asthma and exercise

Becoming breathless is something which can happen to nearly everyone when they exercise. But whereas most people get their breath back quite quickly, children with asthma become more breathless and wheezy.

Running over long distances, e.g. cross-country, causes particular problems, while swimming causes the least. Because exercise-induced asthma is mainly caused by spasm in the muscles around the airways, reliever (bronchodilator) medicines usually provide the best treatment.

Ideally, children should take this form of treatment ten minutes before they exercise, and again if they start to get wheezy.

It is healthier for a child to take some exercise with the help of an inhaler, than to wait on the sidelines and not exercise at all. Encourage your child to be active and to participate in sport. Asthma should not prohibit him or her from leading a normal life and taking part in all school activities.

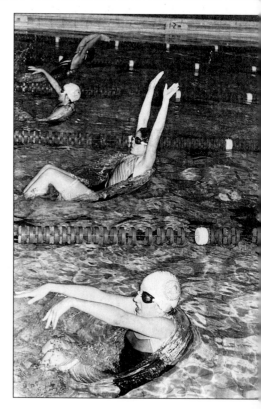

Asthma and school

If your child is diagnosed as having asthma and is starting at a new school, or changing classes and teachers within his or her school, it is always a good idea to tell the school and the class teacher about his asthma and current treatment. There are several good reasons for this:

● To allow the child easy access to his medication. It should not be locked away in a medicine cabinet or the school office. It should be available if he starts wheezing or has an asthma attack. It is distressing for him and could even be dangerous if there is a delay in taking medication. Some schools have a policy of locking up medication, but a child should have his reliever inhaler close at hand at all times.

● To enable the teaching staff to remind a child to take his medicine, e.g. before exercise. Children sometimes forget or feel embarrassed about using their inhaler in front of their classmates.

● To enable the teachers to remind the child to take his medication with him on school outings.

● To understand why a child might be often absent with chest problems.

● To let the school know what to do in the event of an asthma attack.

● To explain to the school the importance of taking preventer medicine on a regular basis as directed by the child's doctor, even if this falls in the middle of the school day.

● Always leave the school a telephone number where you can be contacted in an emergency.

● Science teachers should be aware that certain fumes from experiments can be an allergic trigger and cause problems for some children.

● Some teachers find that they may need to remove pets from the classroom, e.g. guinea pigs, hamsters and rabbits, if they cause wheezing in children.

Tip: Give your child's teacher a written list of the medicines he is taking and when he should have them. Explain how and why his asthma attacks occur and what can be done to prevent and treat them. You could also write down an action plan in the event of an attack.

Sports lessons

Some children suffer from exercise-induced asthma and may need to take a dose of their reliever medicine before they start exercising. A five to ten-minute warm-up before playing games will also help.

Children may sometimes feel awkward and uneasy about joining in with their classmates in PE and games lessons, especially if it makes them wheezy or they have to use their inhaler first. However, they should be encouraged to participate as the fitter they are, the better equipped they will be to cope with an asthma attack. Also,

continued on page 52

Children, allergy and asthma

Asthma and school

continued from page 51

they may become isolated and shunned by their peers if they sit out games lessons and don't join in. Parents and teachers can help children to enjoy sport and to become more confident about exercise. They can also point out that there are top sports people who suffer from asthma and have still gone on to win in their competitive sport, e.g. Ian Botham and Adrian Moorhouse.

Note: if a child becomes wheezy and out of breath during a games lesson, he should never be forced to continue. He should stop immediately and be treated promptly. Likewise, if he is allergic to pollen, he may have to take special care when playing games outside in the summer term.

Dealing with an asthma attack

It is helpful for your child's teachers to know how they can help if your child has an attack. Most children know from experience what to do and can probably handle the situation themselves. However, in the case of young children or a severe attack, they may need help from a teacher.
1 The child should take his reliever medicine promptly. It should be inhaled properly to open up the narrowed airways.
2 Always stay calm and try to reassure the child. Encourage him to breathe slowly and deeply. It may be helpful if he sits upright or leans forward slightly. Don't lie him down on his back. Talk to him calmly and try to take his mind off the attack. You could offer him a glass of warm water to drink if his mouth becomes very dry. If necessary, loosen the top button on his shirt around his neck.
3 After the attack, it is best if he continues with his lessons and normal activities as soon as possible, rather than being excused lessons to lie down and rest.

When to summon help

You should call a doctor or an ambulance if:
● After five to ten minutes the reliever medicine has no effect.
● The child is becoming exhausted and distressed, and is unable to talk.
● You have any doubts whatsoever about the condition of the child.

Note: children sometimes play with their friends' inhalers and spray them around. Obviously, this should be discouraged but they will not come to any harm.

Exercise and asthma

Exercise is good for everyone, even if they have asthma and physical exertion can cause wheezing, chest tightness or breathlessness. Exercise is a common trigger for many children with asthma, yet it does not mean that they have to stop exercising and give up a sport they enjoy. Modern treatments are very effective, and now they can participate in almost any sport. In fact, there are many top sportsmen and women who suffer from asthma but it has not hindered them in their careers – for example, Ian Botham, the cricketer, and Olympic swimmer Adrian Moorhouse.

Exercise-induced asthma

Wheezing, coughing and chest tightness during or after exercise are common symptoms. They are most obvious within a minute of stopping, may worsen over the next few minutes, and may last for up to 30 minutes. During the pollen season, on cold, dry days, or if you have just had a cold, the chances of developing exercise-induced asthma are increased.

Your doctor can diagnose this form of asthma by studying peak flow measurements taken before and after exercise.

Prevention and treatment

Your child can take medicine before exercise to prevent or reduce the symptoms. Your doctor may advise the use of his or her reliever inhaler before exercising instead of when the symptoms appear; or that sodium cromoglycate is taken just before exercising.

Whose asthma, whose medicine?

Using medicines to prevent any asthma symptoms is the best way to get back to normal. However, it is tempting for anyone, child or adult, to feel they are cured if the preventive medicine is working properly. This leads them to get lax about using medicines, or even to stop them altogether. Older children may argue that it is their asthma and they know it best.

Cutting down on treatment can lead to a subtle loss of performance which is easy to miss, and there is the increased risk of a sudden asthma attack. At the same time, it is not always necessary to take drugs at the same level and you can sympathise with any youngsters who would like to take lower doses of a drug.

In fact, just as treatments can be stepped up when your child's asthma is bad, they can also be reduced when it is under better

Children, allergy and asthma

control. Discuss with your doctor whether the time has come to reduce your child's medication.

If the doses are reduced, peak flow monitoring will help you or your child to check the effects of this.

You may also be worried that you don't know how much treatment your child is taking while away from you. If so, you could ask for your child to be switched to a dry powder device, which allows you better to see if more of the drug has been used than is usual.

Some children notice side effects with their preventer medicines, e.g. salbutamol (Ventolin) can cause shaky hands, while terbutaline (Bricanyl) may make the legs feel weak and tired. In this case, they may find it preferable to use terbutaline when working in the classroom, and salbutamol when running on the school field.

Passive smoking

Other people's cigarette smoke poses even more of a problem for asthmatic children than it does for adults with asthma.

Smoking in pregnancy can affect the developing baby, making it more likely to produce the antibodies associated with allergy – and thus more likely to react to different common allergens.

Remember when exercising:

- Breathing in large amounts of cool, dry air on cold days can trigger exercise-induced athma and wheezing. So avoid running outside on cold winter days.
- Short bursts of exercise are less likely to induce asthma than longer spells.
- Exercising in warm, moist air seldom causes asthma, e.g. in indoor swimming pools.
- You are less likely to trigger an attack if you exercise with arms or legs alone.
- If you suffer from hayfever avoid exercising on days when the pollen count is high and could trigger an attack.
- In team games, playing in a less active position could make all the difference between participating and not taking part.
- Children should warm-up before playing games; just sprinting for 30 seconds several times over five to ten minutes will help protect the lungs for up to one hour.
- A child who is physically fit is better able to cope with an asthma attack.
- Children should not be discouraged from taking part in sport just because they have asthma. Physical education treachers in schools should encourage them to participate.
- Children should take their medication before exercising and keep it with them during the class or game.
- A child should not be forced to continue exercising if they say they are too wheezy.

The problems continue once the baby is born. Smoke is particularly harmful for developing lungs and is a powerful irritant which may increase your child's sensitivity to other allergens.

Those children who grow up in smoking households are more likely to be admitted to hospital with chest infections, such as bronchitis and bronchiolitis. Infections can damage the delicate linings of the airways, causing lasting damage to the child.

More than 17,000 children under the age of five are admitted to hospital every year because of the effects of passive smoking.

In the UK it is now estimated that the children of smoking households have twice the risk of developing asthma as the children from non-smoking households.

Research has shown that the symptoms of children with asthma who are exposed to passive smoking are likely to be more severe.

You should avoid smoking near your children, and declare your home a smoke-free zone. For people who have smoked for years, this is easier said than done. However, for the sake of your children's health as well as your own, it is an important step that you should take. Make the decision now to give up smoking. If your partner smokes, try to persuade him or her to stop too. If you find it very difficult, then seek professional medical help. If you are addicted to nicotine in cigarettes, then talk to your doctor about nicotine replacement therapies.

Passive smoking

For many children, their first experience of cigarette smoke is while they are still inside their mother's womb. We now know that smoking during pregnancy increases the likelihood of childhood asthma, and that the babies of mothers who smoke may develop less well in the womb and are born smaller, on average, than the babies of non-smoking mothers.

Children of smoking parents suffer the effects of passive smoking. They breathe in the smoke from smouldering cigarettes and the smoke that is puffed out by their parents. Also they are more likely than the children of non-smokers to develop coughs, colds and chest infections, and twice as likely to develop asthma.

The message is plain: if you smoke, you are putting your child's health at risk. Children with asthma whose parents smoke tend to have more severe symptoms. Their airways are particularly sensitive to cigarette smoke which can cause them to narrow and the linings to become swollen and inflamed. They produce a lot of sticky mucus and this makes them cough a lot.

You should ensure that your child avoids smoky atmospheres and discourage family, friends and guests from smoking in your home. If you cannot stop smoking, go outside for a cigarette instead of smoking inside the house.

Children, allergy and asthma

Asthma and holidays

Both children and adults with asthma can enjoy their holidays with a little forward planning. Here are some useful tips to help you:

● Pack as many tablets and inhalers as you think you will need for the duration of the holiday plus a few extra days.

● Ask your doctor's advice on drawing up a treatment plan.

● Some inhalers do not work effectively in hot, humid conditions so you may need a different model.

● Find out how to get medical help at your holiday destination.

● If you are taking a nebuliser abroad, check the voltage.

● Remember that taking regular preventer medicine can help you avoid most problems

and enjoy your holiday with confidence. Work out what triggers your asthma and avoid those triggers while you are on holiday.

Your medical pack

You should pack the following items. If you are flying, pack them in your carry-on luggage rather than your suitcase which

In the UK the National Asthma Campaign organises special activity holidays for young people aged between seven and 30 with asthma, eczema or both. Under supervision, they join in activities, form new friendships and develop self-confidence. Every group is accompanied by experienced helpers, including a doctor.

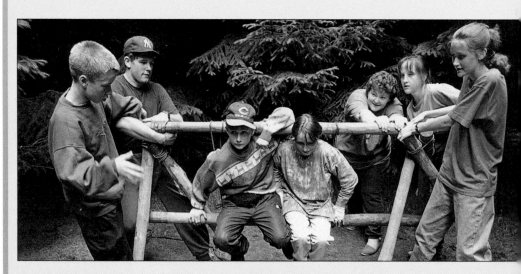

uld get lost or stolen. It is a sensible idea
iyway, to have your medication to hand
st in case you need it during the flight.
  Reliever and preventer medicines.
  Asthma management plan.
  Peak flow meter.
  Aerosol reliever inhaler.
  Steroid tablets for emergencies.
  Emergency action plan.
is also helpful to pack a disposable plastic
 foam coffee cup that can be used as a
mporary spacer in an emergency. Make a
ole in the bottom to fit over the inhaler
outhpiece. You can use this to take puffs
 your reliever medicine. Your doctor will
lvise you on this.

Vhat sort of holiday?

here is no single best sort of holiday for
eople with asthma. People have different
iggers and personal preferences. However,
ie following information may be useful:

ir travel: check with the airline whether
ebulisers are kept on board and book your
eat in advance so that it is well away from
ie smoking section. If possible, on long-
aul flights, choose an airline that has
anned smoking. Ask your travel agent for
dvice on this.

amping and caravanning: these holidays
ring you into contact with pollen, dust
om crops and animals although house dust
iites are less. Avoid camp fire smoke and
arly morning cold air. Ensure that your

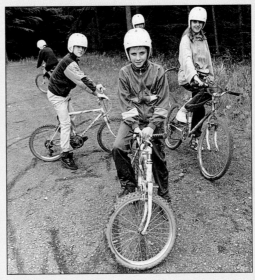

bedding is clean, well-aired and that your
tent has a sewn-in ground sheet.

Climate: generally, warmth is better than
intense heat. High humidity can cause
problems for asthmatics as can dry, dusty
places and desents.

Cruises: these can be a good idea as there
are no pets or pollen, and most ships are
well equipped for medical care, often with a
doctor in attendance.

Skiing holidays: some people find cold
weather beneficial whereas it triggers
symptoms in others. Skiing can be strenuous
so you must take adequate medication with
you. However, house dust mites do not live
above the snow-line.

Children, allergy and asthma

Breastfeeding

Despite the investment of millions of pounds in research, the babymilk manufacturers have been unable to come up with a formula which is as good for human babies as human breastmilk. Breastfeeding for the first six months appears to help prevent infants from becoming allergic to cow's milk, and also helps them avoid the allergic skin condition, eczema. A mother with asthma may pass on a tendency to allergies, rather than asthma itself, to her children. This provides one more reason to breastfeed your baby. However, there is as yet no evidence that breastfeeding will protect your baby against developing asthma, nor will inhaled medicine be present in your breast milk.

Steroids and growth

Children with severe or uncontrolled asthma are likely to be shorter and thinner than others of the same age. The natural hormone which makes children grow is released in bursts during sleep and exercise. If your child is losing sleep and unable to exercise because of asthma, this will also slow down growth. Children with bad asthma often burn up calories from the food they eat faster, and unless they have gargantuan appetites this may also hold back their growth. Once their asthma is brought under control, many children catch up with their peer group.

All this means that uncontrolled asthma can affect a child's growth and development. Unfortunately there is some evidence that long courses of high-dose steroid tablets which are used to control asthma may also limit a child's growth.

However, these long courses should only be used when asthma is indeed severe, e.g. when the child's life might be at risk.

The use of steroids, whether inhaled or in tablet form, should always be carefully monitored, so that children never receive more than is needed to keep their symptoms at bay.

Doctors believe the benefits of controlling asthma with steroids outweigh the risks that growth may be limited. They argue that once the child's asthma is controlled, they are likely to catch up with their peers.

These decisions are difficult, and you and your child have the right to expect the issues to be fully discussed. If you are worried about the steroid drugs that are being prescribed for your child, talk to your doctor about your fears. He will be able to put the case for and against their use, and hopefully allay your fears. More information about steroids is given in Chapter Five.

Chapter five

Drug treatments

Mention asthma treatments, and most people immediately think of the little puffers (aerosol inhalers) which can be carried round in the pocket. In fact, pocket-sized puffers are still the most common way of taking asthma treatments. However, the contents of the inhalers and the way in which they are used has changed.

Until ten years ago, people with asthma relied solely on reliever medicines such as salbutamol (Ventolin) in order to keep their symptoms under control. Now anyone who needs to use a reliever medicine more than once a day is advised to use a preventive treatment as well. If the preventive treatment

proves effective, the symptoms of asthma may be controlled so effectively that the reliever treatment is hardly needed.

Whenever possible, asthma medications are prescribed so that they can be inhaled. This allows the minimum possible dose of the drug to be used because the active ingredient is drawn directly into the airways, just where it is needed.

If a drug is swallowed, a great deal of it is absorbed in other parts of the body, or it is broken down in the liver. This means that doses need to be higher, with a greater risk of side effects. These are explained in more detail later in this chapter.

Aims of treatment

The aims of asthma treatment are to enable the person with asthma to:
● Lead a full, active life.
● Take part in sporting activity (although cross-country running in the winter may not be an option).
● Lose no time from school or work.
● Be free of night-time symptoms.
● Keep lung function as normal as possible.

It is important to be clear about the

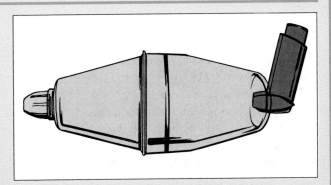

difference between preventer and reliever medicines because they work in completely different ways.

Drug treatments

Preventive treatment

These are anti-inflammatory drugs which damp down the swelling and reduce the mucus in the airways. The aim is not only to reduce the symptoms, but also to minimize the damage which occurs to airways which are almost constantly inflamed and twitchy (hypersensitive).

Most of the preventive treatments are derived from corticosteroids – known as steroids for short. These are quite different from the sex hormones (anabolic steroids) which are abused by some body-builders and athletes. Nevertheless, corticosteroids do

Inhaling steroids is the safest method of taking them as the drug goes straight to the lungs and only a small dose is needed. They can be breathed in using a puffer(aerosol inhaler), sometimes with a spacer, a dry powder inhaler or a nebuliser(as shown here).

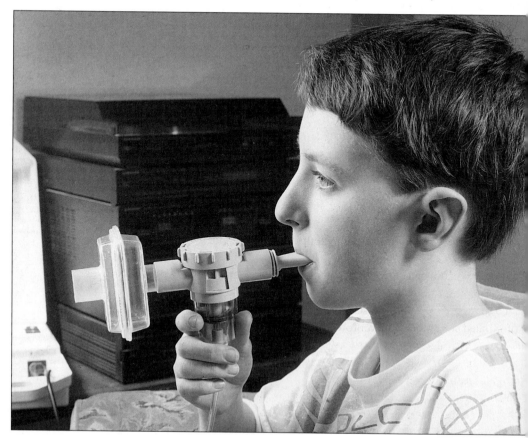

Steroid treatment for asthma

Corticosteroids, the sort that are used to treat asthma, are made artificially by the big pharmaceutical companies. They reduce the amount of inflammation, swelling and mucus in the airways and thereby help prevent breathing difficulties. There are three ways in which you can take them:

● To prevent asthma – by inhaling them direct into the lungs.

● To relieve acute attacks and control severe asthma – by swallowing them in the form of steroid tablets.

● To treat acute, severe attacks – by a doctor or nurse injecting them.

Inhaled steroids

These are the most common preventer for adults, although not for children for whom steroids are prescribed only if sodium cromoglycate is not effective. When inhaled, steroids do not relieve an asthma attack. They need to be taken over a period of time to slowly reduce inflammation and mucus in the airways and it may take up to two weeks before you notice the benefits. It is important to take them every day whether you are getting asthma symptoms or not. If you catch a cold, your doctor may recommend that you increase the amount of inhaled steroid for added protection.

Side effects: there are very few although you may become hoarse or get the odd minor mouth and throat infection(see page 63). Using a spacer device reduces the risk of side effects.

Steroid tablets

These are prescribed either as short courses to relieve severe, acute athma, or as long courses to control chronic asthma on a day-to-day basis. Steroid tablets work quickly – after a few hours – and may be needed if your asthma worsens.

Short courses: these may last up to two weeks for adults; three to four days for a child. They have few side effects, although some people report a temporary increase in appetite and small weight gain. Children may become more excitable than usual. It is advisable not to take more than two or three courses a year.

Long courses: few people need to take long courses of steroid tablets to control their asthma. In these cases, only the smallest possible dose is prescribed. If taken over a period of months, they can have serious side effects, including weight gain, thinning of the bones(osteoporosis) and increased blood pressure. A long course is rarely given to children and then only every other day to minimize unpleasant side effects. On a dose of 5mg per day or less, side effects are minimal.

Injecting steroids

Injections are used only to treat acute, severe asthma and are performed by a doctor or nurse. However, they do not work faster than tablets and are usually used only if the patient is unwell or sick.

Drug treatments

have some side effects, which are discussed in more detail below.

Inhaled steroids are usually taken twice a day; and you may find it easier to remember if you take them just before cleaning your teeth in the morning and evening. Rinsing your mouth out at this time helps reduce the risk of getting oral thrush, or a sore throat, which are both occasional but annoying side effects of inhaled steroids.

Steroids can take up to 14 days before they work their full effects so don't expect to see results straight away.

The commonest inhaled steroids include beclomethasone dipropionate (Becotide, Becloforte, AeroBec), budesonide (Pulmicort) and fluticasone propionate (Flixotide).

There are some preventer treatments which do not contain steroids, e.g. sodium cromoglycate (Intal) and nedocromil sodium (Tilade Mint). They also work by reducing inflammation, but are not always as effective as steroid treatments.

Sodium cromoglycate is often used as a preventer treatment for children, but it is less useful in treating adults. It also works well as a reliever medicine in the treatment of any exercise-induced asthma.

The aim of modern treatments is to get asthma completely under control using preventer treatments alone. When this is achieved, it is tempting to assume that you are cured, and to simply stop taking the medication. However, this is not advisable as it exposes you to the risk of a sudden, uncontrolled asthma attack.

If your disease has been well controlled for several months, then you could ask your doctor if you can 'step down' by reducing your dose of preventer medicine. You shoul always do this under medical supervision, and, preferably, monitor your peak flow to check that the asthma is not about to flare up again.

When the standard dose inhalers fail to control asthma, a higher dose version is used. If this is also unsuccessful, doctors ma prescribe steroid tablets, usually in the form of the drug prednisolone. This may be given as a short course to relieve the inflammation which has caused a severe asthma attack, or in smaller, daily doses. A typical child's shor course may last three to four days, while adults may require a longer course of steroic for about two weeks.

Many doctors now give patients a short course of steroid tablets to be taken when their asthma gets worse, e.g. an increase in night-time waking, or falling peak flow readings.

Side effects from steroid preventers

Inhaled steroids are a very efficient treatmen for asthma, and for many people they can represent the difference between being ill and living a normal life. Doctors confidently prescribe them because they are convinced that the benefits vastly outweigh the risks.

However, many people have a knee-jerk reaction to steroids on the lines of "steroids me? You must be joking."

This extreme response may lead doctors to err on the cautious side, and play down the side effects of steroids rather than take the risk that patients will refuse to take them

Research shows that failure to take these prescribed steroids is extremely common. Patients with asthma seldom confront their doctors about their side-effect worries, and they simply tend to leave the steroid inhaler unused in its box.

Inhaled preparations give a much lower dose of steroid than tablets because the drug goes straight to the airways rather than being broken down in the body. Nevertheless, a little of the inhaled steroid is inevitably swallowed and thereby absorbed into the bloodstream. However, there is no medical evidence that low-dose inhaled steroids cause any major side effects.

People who take inhaled steroids have an increased risk of getting thrush infections of the throat and mouth, hoarseness, and coughing. Rinsing the mouth after taking the drug, using one of the spacers described below and eating live yoghurt all help to reduce these unwanted side effects.

Sometimes the standard dose in steroid inhalers is not enough and higher strengths of the drug are required.

Spacer devices (explained on page 68) help to reduce the risks of steroids being absorbed into the body. They do this by making it easier to inhale the drug. This, in turn, reduces the amount of steroid which is deposited in the back of the throat and then swallowed and absorbed by the body.

Nevertheless, an increased dose does carry an increased risk of side effects. This risk is, however, less than with the alternative steroid tablets, and is certainly less risky than experiencing a severe and uncontrolled asthma attack.

A short course of steroid tablets may cause a slight weight gain and even mood changes, especially in children. However, the risks of two or three short courses in a single year are considered to be low.

Longer courses of steroids, taken over many months, can cause some weight gain, the thinning of the bones (osteoporosis), increased blood pressure, stomach ulcers and an increased risk that diabetes will occur in people who are already predisposed to develop it. The magnitude of the risk from steroids depends on the dose. Side effects become more likely on doses which exceed 5mg a day.

Steroid tablets are usually taken in the prescribed dose once a day only, rather than several times a day, to reduce the side effects. Sometimes they are taken on alternate days.

Patients who need high-dose tablets may feel that they are between a rock and a hard place. If asthma is very severe, and making normal life impossible, or indeed if it is life-threatening, they may decide they have no choice but to take the drugs.

Summary

Steroids are very good at preventing asthma. They are taken in three ways:
- By inhaling them.
- By swallowing them(tablets).
- By injecting them.

Drug treatments

Warning

WARNING: While artificial steroids are being taken, the body reduces its natural production of steroid hormones. A sudden cessation of treatment leaves an individual unprepared to deal with the stress caused by an accident, infection or surgery.

For this reason it is dangerous to suddenly stop taking steroids (this applies only to the longer courses, and not to the short courses or the inhaled steroids).

People who are currently taking high-dose steroids, or have taken them in the previous two years, need to carry special warning cards in case they are injured or suddenly taken ill. The cards alert doctors to the fact that the individuals concerned will need extra steroids while they are receiving treatment.

Reliever medicines

Most of the reliever medicines are based on adrenaline, the hormone produced naturally in the body at times of stress. A rush of adrenaline allows us to think clearly and act quickly in a crisis, and it is often known as the 'fight or flight' hormone.

One of its effects is to open the airways. Drugs in this category are known as adrenergic bronchodilators or beta-agonists or beta-stimulants.

They are taken at the first sign of any breathing difficulties, when peak monitor readings are lowered and before exercise, and they are effective for about four hours. If you need to take your reliever medicine more often than this, it is quite safe to do so. However, this is a sign that your asthma is getting out of control and you should consult a doctor. Two of the commonest reliever medicines are salbutamol (Ventolin) and terbutaline (Bricanyl).

Long acting relievers

When asthma and coughing occur despite the use of a preventer and reliever medicine, or if you have troublesome asthma in the middle of the night (nocturnal asthma), your

Side effects of sodium cromoglycate preventers

Sodium cromoglycate (Intal) can sometimes cause irritation and coughing. Taking reliever medicine a few minutes beforehand seems to help. Intal is strongly protective against many allergies, and you should not stop it suddenly because you could suddenly lose the protection the drug offers. If you come off Intal, you should tail off the dose over the course of a week or so.

octor may suggest a longer acting reliever rug. Their effects can last up to 12 hours.

These drugs include two inhaled ones: xitropium (Oxivent) and salmeterol 3erevent). Another long-acting reliever, heophylline (Slo-Phyllin and Uniphyllin), is urrently only available in tablet form.

Drugs in this group work in a similar vay to the other relievers, and they do not 2duce the inflammation in the airways. For nis reason, they cannot be taken instead of ne anti-inflammatory preventive treatments.

ide effects of relievers

ny drug which is strong enough to have an ffect on symptoms carries the risks of side ffects as well. There is a choice of asthma rugs in all categories of treatment, so if one type disagrees with you, there is usually an alternative for you to try.

The main side effects of beta-agonist reliever medicines, such as salbutamol (Ventolin) and terbutaline (Bricanyl), are a trembling of the muscles, particularly in the hands.

Relievers in the anti-cholinergic drug group, such as ipratropium (Atrovent) and oxitropium (Oxivent), can cause a dry mouth, blurred vision, difficulties in passing urine and constipation. Theophylline-type drugs can lead to disorders of the heart rhythm, e.g. rapid heart rate and irregular heart beats. Other side effects may include flushing, nettle rash, nausea, vomiting, diarrhoea, dizziness, vertigo, light-headedness, nervousness, headaches, irritability, restlessness and over-excitability.

Drugs that can cause asthma

You may not realise that some drugs can actually cause asthma, notably the following:

● Aspirin and non-steroidal anti-inflammatory drugs(NSAIDS).

● Drugs that may be prescribed for high blood pressure and which may be used as eye drops for people with high tension in the eye.

The so-called 'Beta-Blocker' drugs are rarely used for treating asthmatics. In some people, their use can give rise to mild asthma, the first tell-tale sign being a cough. If your doctor is treating you for high blood pressure, remind him that you are asthmatic so that he can choose the best drug to treat your condition safely.

If you are asthmatic and aspirin sensitive, beware of taking over-the-counter remedies for colds and rheumatism that contain aspirin. If you are unsure of which drugs are aspirin free(contain no acetyl salicylic acid), then ask your doctor or the pharmacist for advice. Paracetamol can usually be taken with no rise in asthmatic symptoms.

Drug treatments

Inhalers, spacers and nebulisers

Your choice of inhaler is not simply a matter of cost, or of preference. Many people are unable to get their asthma under control simply because they are taking the right drugs in the wrong way.

If you are uncertain whether you are truly inhaling your drugs (you may, for instance, just be swallowing them), then ask for some guidance. Your family doctor or asthma nurse will be happy to help you check whether your technique is right.

Some people just need a little guidance, e.g. they are pressing the spray too soon, or not breathing in for long enough. Others simply cannot get on with one type of device, and yet will be much happier with another. There follows the various choices which are available in the UK to most National Health Service patients:

Aerosol sprays

Also known as puffers, these are used for both reliever and preventer treatments. The medicine is mixed into a liquid and forced under pressure into a small canister.

Once it is activated, the mixer liquid

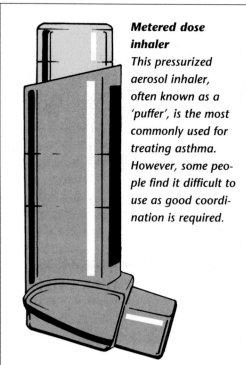

Metered dose inhaler
This pressurized aerosol inhaler, often known as a 'puffer', is the most commonly used for treating asthma. However, some people find it difficult to use as good coordination is required.

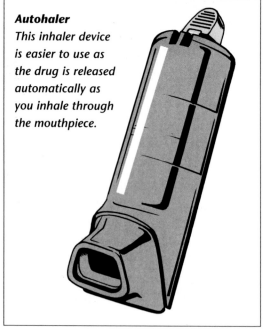

Autohaler
This inhaler device is easier to use as the drug is released automatically as you inhale through the mouthpiece.

quickly evaporates, leaving behind the active ingredient to be breathed in. Each time the canister is pushed down, a measured (metered) dose of the drug is released. It usually takes about 30 seconds to recharge the spray ready for the next dose.

The Autohaler is useful for people who are unable to co-ordinate pushing down the canister with an in-breath. Instead, it works automatically as you breathe in.

Powder inhalers

These make it easier to keep a check on how much medicine has been taken – and how much is left (something that is often hard to gauge on a standard aerosol). The medicine itself comes in dry powder form, contained in a capsule. As the device is activated, the capsule is broken allowing the powder to be inhaled. Some devices have the powder inside a disk or compartment.

Turbohaler
This is easy to use and delivers asthma drugs in a dry powder form.

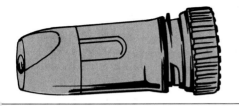

Rotahaler, Spinhaler and Diskhaler
The rotahaler together with the Spinhaler and Diskhaler, this also gives the drug in dry powder form. You can monitor the number of doses taken with the Diskhaler.

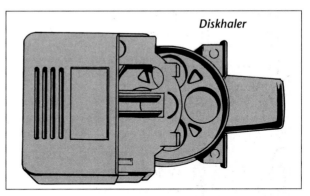

Diskhaler

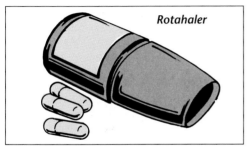

Rotahaler

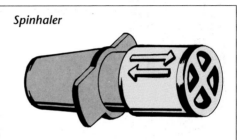

Spinhaler

Drug treatments

The Aerochamber

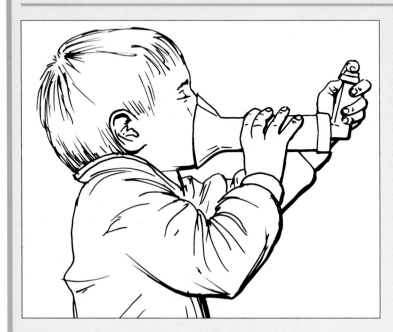

The Aerochamber is smaller than most spacers and is particularly suitable for children who cannot use the mouthpiece of a spacer. It fits all inhalers snugly and is available in baby, child and adult sizes with a mask.

Using a spacer

Spacers deliver medicine more efficiently than an inhaler alone. They are easy to use: the inhaler is shaken, put into the spacer device and then squirted. You have up to five seconds to take one large breath in. However, if you are short of breath, you can just breathe in and out normally rather than taking one big breath. Spacers are used for the following reasons:

● To give a higher dose of medicine during asthma attacks.

● To give the propellant time to evaporate before inhaling the medicine.

● To give inhaled medicines to small children who cannot use the mouthpiece of an inhaler. Some children learn to do so between two and four years old.

● To give inhaled medicines to the elderly.

● To diminish the risk of steroids being absorbed into the body, and side effects such as minor mouth and throat infections(thrush).

Spacers

These are largish canisters which are attached to a standard aerosol spray. When the aerosol is activated, the drug is trapped into the spacer which is placed over the mouth and nose as you breathe in. This reduces the chances of swallowing the drug instead of inhaling it, and is also useful for those people (including children) who have problems co-ordinating breathing and the action of an aerosol inhaler.

Coffee cup spacer

In an emergency, if there is no spacer available, you can make a substitute one with a disposable coffee cup. Use a plastic or foam cup and make a hole in the base which is large enough to fit the inhaler. Using the cup as a mask, squirt the inhaler into your lungs. Inevitably, this is not as effective as the real thing and some of the medicine will be lost. However, it is effective and some of the medicine will reach your lungs.

Nebulisers

Nebulisers work by forcing air or oxygen through a liquid preparation of the drug, thereby producing a fine mist.

Nebulisers are mainly used for taking large doses of reliever medicines when asthma is severe. However, many people find that using a spacer is more convenient, and just as effective as a nebuliser.

Nebulisers are also used to deliver doses of reliever and preventer medicines to children who are too young to use other devices, such as inhalers.

Children and spacers

Young children should use a spacer with a face mask to fit their aerosol puffer. They may be unable to use the mouthpiece of an inhaler until they are about four years old, and the spacer ensures that the medicine given reaches their lungs instead of their mouths or throats.

Tips for babies

● Use it when the baby is asleep – just hold the spacer and mask over his face and he will breathe in the treatment.

● To get the baby used to the feel of the mask, gently stroke his cheek with it.

● When using the spacer, hold the baby with his arms wrapped up.

● Even if your baby is crying, you can gently hold the mask over his face and the medicine will still be inhaled.

Tips for toddlers

● Show your toddler how to use the spacer and mask.

● Decorate it with colourful stickers and make it into a toy.

● Count aloud as your child takes breaths from the spacer, and make it a counting game.

● Pretend that the spacer is a strange-looking trumpet.

Drug treatments

Nebulisers

There are two types of nebuliser: the jet nebuliser and the ultrasonic nebuliser. They are both effective means of getting medicine into the lungs safely. They should only be used if recommended by your doctor, as follows:

For treating small children
A spacer with a mask is best for babies, but a nebuliser may be used by young children to inhale preventer medicine.

● **For treating severe persistent asthma**
A nebuliser can give larger doses of reliever medicine than an inhaler and may be more effective for people with severe asthma. Some may find that they also need a nebulised steroid preventer.

● **For emergency treatment**
Again, because a nebuliser can give a larger dose than an inhaler, it is used to administer reliever medicine to bring rapid relief in a severe attack of asthma. Some people benefit from having their own home nebuliser or portable model, but most asthmatics can control their asthma without one.

Should you have a nebuliser?
You can buy a nebuliser but before you make such a purchase, talk it over with your doctor to see if you really need one. He will be able to advise you on which type to choose if it is necessary for you to have one. In the UK, hospital consultants can prescribe a nebuliser in some cases, and some hospitals will loan them to patients. Electric nebulisers are quite expensive but you can purchase a cheaper foot pump model. If you are considering this option, bear in mind that in the event of an asthma attack, you will need somebody to work the foot pump for you.

Preventer medicines
The following medicines can be used in a nebuliser:
● Sodium cromoglycate
● Budesonide
● Beclomethasone

Reliever medicines
The following medicines can be used in a nebuliser:
● Salbutamol
● Terbutaline
● Fenoterol
● Ipratropium bromide

How to use a nebuliser
1 Plug the pump into a mains supply socket, and then connect the tubing to the nebuliser.
2 Pour the medicine into the drug chamber and attach the mouthpiece or mask.
3 Place the mouthpiece in your mouth or put on the mask.
4 Switch on the compressor and a fine mist of medicine will appear in the mask.
5 Breathe normally. The treatment is

omplete, when the nebuliser starts to plutter.

fter use, switch off the machine and sconnect the tubing. Clean the nebuliser nd mouthpiece thoroughly. Make sure that ie tubing is dry before putting it away.

ote: While you use the nebuliser, sit in a nair or on a bed in a well supported osition.

nportant guidelines

you are using a nebuliser at home, make re that you follow your doctor's advice on ow to manage your asthma and understand hen and how to use the nebuliser. Here are me guidelines to help you:

● Ask your doctor how to assemble and use your nebuliser correctly and to explain to you how it works. You should also find out how to keep it clean, and about repairing and servicing it and replacing parts.

● Ask your doctor to write down detailed instructions on your medicines, e.g. which you should use, how often and in what dosage.

● Your doctor may give you a self-management plan, which will help you to recognise the warning signs of an asthma attack and when to start using the nebuliser.

● If the nebuliser does not relieve the attack, it is important to summon medical help immediately. Do not delay.

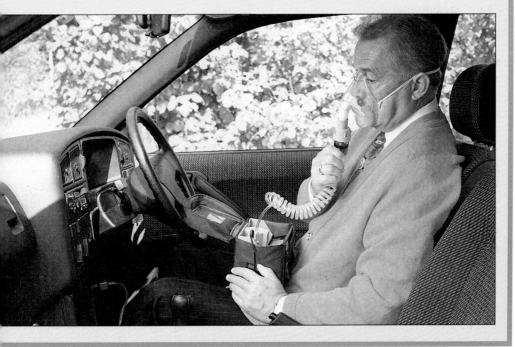

Drug treatments

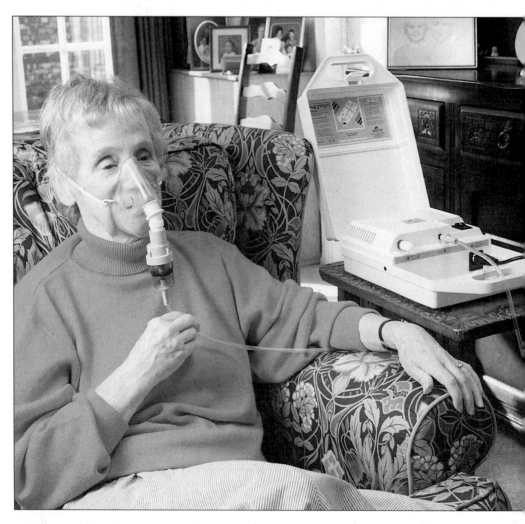

A nebuliser breaks up a liquid medicine into a mist of tiny droplets which can be inhaled through a mouthpiece or mask straight into the lungs. The liquid medicine is housed within a small cointainer in the nebuliser unit, and air oxygen is blown through it to create a mist. T is achieved by means of an electric air pump, even a hand or foot pump in some models.

Chapter six
Complementary therapies

Asthma can be a lifelong condition, and may involve lifelong drug taking. Many people wonder if gentler, more natural therapies would be a healthier alternative.

However, medical evidence suggests that giving up asthma drugs can allow further damage to inflamed airways. In severe cases this could lead to increased disablement, e.g. inability to walk up stairs or leave the house on a cold day and possibly even death from an uncontrolled attack of asthma.

While only a tiny minority of people with asthma are at risk of actually dying from the condition, it is not always possible to predict who these high-risk people are.

The word 'complementary' means forming a satisfactory or balanced whole. This is quite different from 'alternative',

Acupuncture

This is a form of traditional Chinese medicine in which special fine acupuncture needles are inserted at specific points on the body, usually in conjunction with herbal remedies. The Chinese believe that good health is dependent on achieving an internal balance of energies and harmony in which the organs of the body interact. In their view, an asthma attack is linked to deficiencies of energy in the airways in the lungs, which become blocked by mucus.

Acupuncture can be used to readjust the balance of energies and encourage the energy to flow through the airways. There is evidence that acupuncture can relieve wheezing, and the benefit is similar to that obtained from using a bronchodilator aerosol. It has also been demonstrated to protect against exercise-induced asthma and to soothe twitchy airways.

Very fine needles are inserted by the acupuncturist at points on the energy channels to restore the flow of energy and restore normal breathing. The needles are stimulated, usually by gentle twisting, so that the energy will pass into the channel and overcome any obstruction in the airways.

Many people have benefited from acupuncture as a preventive treatment on a short-term basis. However, there is as yet insufficient evidence that repeated and regular treatments bring long-term benefits.

Complementary therapies

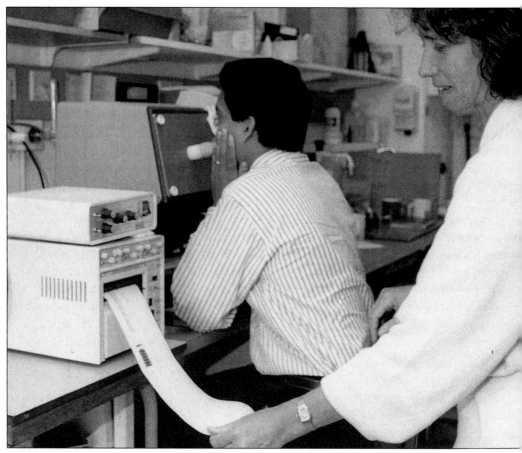

which implies a choice between one thing or another. Some research findings do suggest that certain complementary therapies can be effective for treating asthma when combined with conventional medicine.

For example, acupuncture has been shown to have some mild beneficial effects on wheezing symptoms.

Hypnosis, relaxation and yoga have all proved to be helpful in relieving stress, which is an important asthma trigger.

Unfortunately, people who are stressed

Important medical research is being carried out into the causes and treatment of asthma, and conventional drug treatment is still the safest and most effective method of treatment. In contrast there has been little research and rigorous testing of complementary therapies.

are often too strung out to persist with such treatments, or insist that their lives are hectic and they don't have the time. Dealing with stress has to include setting aside time for yourself and sticking to this appointment as gorously as to any others in your day.

Some people believe that homeopathy is seful in the treatment of the milder cases of sthma. If you are considering homeopathy s an alternative to drug treatments, it is ssential that you consult a homeopathic octor who is also medically qualified.

Osteopathy may also help to improve nuscle spasms in the chest wall. For more nformation turn to page 79 at the back of ne book.

Vast sums of money are being spent on eveloping and testing new asthma drugs. ome of this money is poured into valuable nedical research, which might not otherwise e carried out.

The people who market complementary nerapies seldom carry out this kind of esearch and, as a result, their treatments are rarely subjected to any rigorous tests or long follow up. This makes it difficult to judge their true effectiveness or to make confident recommendations about them.

Another difficulty in assessing some complementary therapies lies in the 'placebo effect'. This occurs when people get better because they are convinced that the treatment they are taking – no matter how bizarre – is going to work for them.

Whenever a new drug is tested against dummy pills (placebos), a large number of people taking the dummy pills will report an improvement in their condition.

The difference between the placebo effect and a treatment which genuinely cures or relieves symptoms is that the placebos are usually short-lasting and have no long-term effects in the treatment of their asthma.

Homeopathy

This approach is sometimes used for the prevention and treatment of asthma. In fact, many medical doctors also practise homeopathy and if you are considering homeopathic treatment it is best to consult a homeopath who is medically qualified.

Homeopathy was devised by a German doctor Hahnemann in the late eighteenth century. He observed that some herbal remedies which could cure a disease could also produce the symptoms of that disease. He developed the homeopathic principle of 'Like cures like', whereby a preparation that can produce the symptoms of a disease is given in a very dilute form to treat and cure the same disease.

Homeopaths believe that the more diluted a remedy is, the more powerful it is in effecting a cure. In the treatment of asthma, there is as yet no evidence that it is an effective alternative therapy and it should not be used instead of conventional drug treatments. However, it can be used to complement the treatment you receive from your doctor, and if you wish to try it you should ask him to recommend a homeopathic physician in your area.

Complementary therapies

Creating a low-allergen garden

Some people who suffer from acute asthma and are allergic to pollen grains and mould spores rarely venture out into their gardens, particularly in the summer months when pollen counts are high. However, there are other allergens at different times of the year that can cause breathing difficulties and wheezing: for instance tree pollen in spring, and weed pollen and mould spores in autumn. Whereas some people are sensitive to just one allergen, others are sensitive to several.

Most people deal with this by staying away from allergens; this often means staying inside with the windows closed, especially mid-morning when pollen is released and rises into the air, and also during the late afternoon and early evening when the air cools and the pollen cloud descends.

It is not possible to create a garden that is free from pollen grains and mould spores, but you can design your own low-allergen garden and take some practical preventive measures when gardening or relaxing in the garden. In 1993 in the UK a specially designed low-allergen garden was on show at the Chelsea Flower Show. It was devised for the National Asthma Campaign in consultation with leading allergists, botanists and professional gardeners who are asthmatic. Here are some useful tips and advice to help you design your own low-allergen garden.

Choosing plants, shrubs and trees

When choosing plants, you should try to avoid the ones that produce wind-carried pollen. Unfortunately, this category includes all grasses, some wild flowers and many trees. It is safer to opt for insect-pollinated plants.

Insect pollinated plants: these include the following:
- Most shrubs with the exception of heavily scented ones like broom, buddleia, caenothus, honeysuckle, jasmine and philadelphus.
- Most showy flowers are pollinated by insects and are suitable to plant. However, again, there are exceptions. If you are pollen sensitive, you may find that the following plants make you wheezy:
- Asters
- Carnations
- Chrysanthemums
- Dahlias
- Daisies
- Pinks
- Sweet Williams

If heavily scented flowers are a problem, especially when cut and brought indoors, you might have to avoid planting the following:
- Daffodils
- Friesias

Hyacinths
Roses which are heavily scented(some
rieties have little scent)
Sweet peas

ees: with the exception of fruit trees,
ost trees are wind-pollinated. If you are
anting young trees, keep them well away
om your house at the other end of the
rden. The trees that often produce allergic
actions include the following:

Ash	● Oak
Birch	● Pine
Elder	● Plane
Hazel	● Sycamore
Horse chestnut	● Willow
Lime	● Yew

Hedges: if possible, you should avoid planting hedges and use fencing, trellis work and shrubs instead. This is because hedges tend to collect pollen from other plants in the garden. When they are cut, clouds of pollen dust are released.

● **Herbs:** these are insect-pollinated plants and are well tolerated by people with asthma and hayfever. Nevertheless, it is a good idea to pick them before they flower. If you dry your own herbs, do this outside in a shed or garage rather than risk introducing any mould spores into your home.

● **Water plants:** these are all safe to plant, but if you have a water garden it might be sensible to forego a fountain. The spray can carry mould spores into the air.

Gardening tips

Always wear a hat to prevent pollen
tting in your hair.

No matter how enthusiastic a gardener
u are, you can do without a compost
ap which is a source of mould spores.

If possible, get somebody else who is not
ergic to cut and prune hedges, and burn
rden rubbish.

If weeding causes problems and makes
u wheeze, consider filling in the gaps
tween plants with ground cover plants.
You can use low-allergen mulch(gravel)
suppress weeds after preparing the soil
low it.

Avoid oranic mulches, e.g. tree bark and

mushroom compost, which are broken down by moulds.

● If mowing the lawn makes you wheezy and short of breath, you may have to get somebody else to do this chore for you. A cylinder mower which collects the grass cuttings is best.

● It is a shame to concrete over your garden, but terraces can look very attractive and can be constructed in natural materials, such as slate and stone to create a nice effect.

It may be necessary to do this if you cannot mow the lawn because of the dust that this releases into the air.

Complementary therapies

A gardener's calender

There are times of the year when it is easier to work in the garden than others. Here is a brief seasonal guide:

Spring
In the northern hemisphere, the pollen season starts in April when the trees blossom. To avoid tree pollens, plant trees away from the house or opt for fruit trees. Grass pollen is usually released from late May onwards.

Summer
Grass pollen continues to be a problem right through the summer months. When the weather is warm and sunny, millions of grass pollen grains are released in the early morning and descend in the evening. To avoid hayfever, work in the garden in the middle of the day. Flowers release their pollens too during the summer months, usually from June to late September. Fungi release their mould spores in damp weather.

Autumn
Early autumn(September) is still a time when pollen counts are relatively high and fungi are active, especially at night.

Winter
The pollen season is over and the fungi lie dormant during the colder winter months.

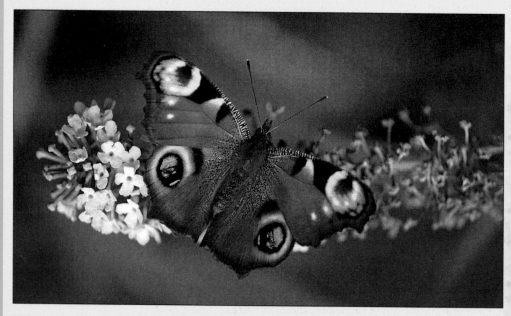

Useful information

e National Asthma Campaign

the UK, the National Asthma Campaign has a full ge of information on asthma. Their helpline is en between 9am and 9pm from Monday to Friday d is staffed by qualified asthma nurses. You can call em on 0345 010203(calls are charged at local rates).

If you want to contact other people with hma, or to support the Campaign's efforts to lp people with asthma lead normal lives, then u can join one of nearly 200 local branches in eat Britain. Details are available by ringing the lpline number listed above.

The National Asthma Campaign is an dependent charity which deals with all aspects of hma and related allergy. It funds research, reads knowledge and provides advice and support people with asthma. If you would like to make a nation and/or receive more information about hma or the National Asthma Campaign, please ite to: **The National Asthma Campaign**
Providence House
Providence Place
London N1 0NT
Tel: 071 226 2260

her useful information

r information on how to safeguard your rights to an air, contact: **Action on Smoking and Health**
Breathing Space Campaign
109 Gloucester Place
London W1H 3PH
r details of the air quality in your locality, you n ring the Department of the Environment's Air ality Information Line: Tel: 0800 556677

you believe that your asthma is occupational, u can apply for compensation from the partment of Social Security. Get a leaflet on cupational asthma from your local DSS office.

For a list of general practitioners with asthma clinics, ring your Community Health Council or Family Health Services Authority. The phone numbers are avilable in your local telephone directory or from the library.
Note: enclose a stamped addressed envelope

Complementary treatment

To get further details of practising homeopathic physicians, write to:
Faculty of Homeopathy
London Homeopathic Hospital
Great Ormond Street
London WC1N 1RJ

British Osteopathic Association
8-10 Boston Place
London NW1 6QH

Overseas useful addresses

Australia
Brian C. Rope
P.O. Box 360, Woden A.C.T. 2606
Tel: 06 2823265

New Zealand
Brenda Wilson
P.O. Box 1459, 7th Floor, Rossmore House
123 Molesworth Street, Wellington
Tel: 04 499 4592

USA
Jennifer Miller
Allergy and Asthma Network/Mothers of Asthmatics Inc.
3554 Chain Bridge Road, Suite 200, Fairfax
Virginia 22030
Tel: (703) 385 4403

Index